# STUTTERING SELF-HELP
# FOR ADULTS

# STUTTERING SELF-HELP
# FOR ADULTS

*By*

**MORRIS VAL JONES, PH.D.**

*Professor Emeritus*
*Department of Speech Pathology and Audiology*
*California State University, Sacramento*
*and*
*Speech Pathologist*
*Robertson Adult Day Health Care Center*
*Sacramento, California*

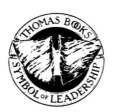

C H A R L E S  C  T H O M A S  •  P U B L I S H E R
*Springfield • Illinois • U.S.A.*

*Published and Distributed Throughout the World by*

CHARLES C THOMAS • PUBLISHER
2600 South First Street
Springfield, Illinois 62794-9265

© *1989 by* CHARLES C THOMAS • PUBLISHER

ISBN 0-398-05568-8

Library of Congress Catalog Card Number: 88-34689

*With* THOMAS BOOKS *careful attention is given to all details of manufacturing
and design. It is the Publisher's desire to present books that are satisfactory as to their
physical qualities and artistic possibilities and appropriate for their particular use.*
THOMAS BOOKS *will be true to those laws of quality that assure a good name
and good will.*

*Printed in the United States of America*
*SC-R-3*

**Library of Congress Cataloging-in-Publication Data**

Jones, Morris Val.
    Stuttering self-help for adults/by Morris Val Jones.
    p.   cm.
Bibliography: p.
    Includes index.
    ISBN 0-398-05568-8
    1. Stuttering—Treatment. 2. Self-care, Health. I. Title.
RC424.J78  1989
616.85'5406—dc19                                              8-34689
                                                                    CIP

*This guidebook about stuttering is dedicated to the four generations of women who have inspired me to keep my shoulder to the wheel . . . and finish it.*

*Gertrude . . . mother*

*Patricia . . . wife*

*Laurie . . . daughter*

*Sabrina . . . granddaughter*

*And then there is Jane (sister-in-law)*

# PREFACE

Stuttering, also known as disfluency or stammering, is an intriguing subarea of speech pathology. This text is designed as a self-help resource for stutterers. No text can replace the therapeutic process based on rapport between clinician and client; my aim is for this book to be helpful as a supplement to clinician-guided therapy.

Charles Van Riper, an international expert in the area of stuttering, believes that the therapist's credibility must be established at the beginning of therapy. The therapist must impress the client with knowledge and clinical skills. Van Riper believes that such a clinician-client relationship is essential throughout the weeks or months of therapy; that, without it, little or no progress toward normal fluency patterns can emerge. Establishing these credentials helps instill the hope that the prognosis is favorable, and that progress toward fluency is possible. This hope motivates active, positive participation, leading to progress.

In line with Van Riper's prescription, I thought it appropriate to establish my credentials as the author of advice for stutterers. My first exposure to stuttering was in an introductory course in speech disorders taught by the late Wendell Johnson at the University of Iowa, one of the first universities in the United States to have a department of speech pathology. Under the leadership of Lee Edward Travis, the University of Iowa became the Mecca for aspiring speech pathologists, producing hundreds of doctorates. Among the outstanding graduates are Charles Van Riper, Wendell Johnson, Dean Williams, Oliver Bloodstein, and, more recently, Edward Conture and Frederick Darley.

I received professional training at Stanford University, where Virgil Anderson was building a viable program in speech pathology. Anderson was a California authority on stuttering as well as being an author of articulation and language development textbooks. His therapeutic approach was eclectic, incorporating elements from such diverse schools of thought as psychology, learning theory, and operant conditioning. He also emphasized the necessity of a specifically tailored therapy program for each client, based on research of the literature, extensive clinical experience, and thorough knowledge of the client's individual needs.

My first professional publication was a translation of the ideas of Leopold Treitel, a German speech pathologist, about therapy for stutterers. Subsequently, I gained extensive practical experience by establishing a speech therapy program in the public schools in Santa Ana, teaching speech pathology at the University level, and being a speech pathologist in a rehabilitation center. My first book, *Speech Correction at Home* (Charles C Thomas, 1959), included a chapter on stuttering. In the ensuing years, I have dealt with hundreds of stutterers, both directly in therapy and indirectly as a supervisor of students with stuttering clients.

For over twenty years, I was a faculty member of the Department of Speech Pathology and Audiology at California State University, Sacramento (CSUS), where my professional assignments included teaching stuttering theory and supervising student therapists. Until 1985, my duties were those of a full-time, tenured full professor; now, semi-retired, I have kept professionally active by working as a speech therapist for the Robertson Adult Day Health Care Center in Sacramento, California. To add to my knowledge, I attend numerous state and national conferences, as well as workshops by leading experts on stuttering such as Hugo Gregory, George Shames, Joseph Sheehan, William Perkins, and Frederick Murray.

When I studied Lloyd Hulit's *Stuttering: In Perspective* (1985), I was reminded of a long-standing controversy among professionals in speech pathology. Is having had a speech defect in a specific subarea, i.e., stuttering, aphasia, laryngectomy, hearing loss, etc., a prerequisite for becoming a therapist in that area? In identifying himself, Hulit writes, "It is important for you to know that I am a stutterer . . . One of my qualifications is that I am a stutterer. I have lived with this speech disorder most of my life, certainly all of the life I can remember." Indeed, some of the most widely known university experts in stuttering have been severe stutterers; these include Charles Van Riper, Joseph Shechen, Wendell Johnson, and Frederick Murray.

Many stuttering therapists have implied that the "condition" is essential to becoming a successful therapist. Since I am not a stutterer and never have been, I was concerned with this assertion. My anxiety was relieved somewhat when Hulit continued, "My experience as a stutterer is the least of my qualifications. It is the understanding of stuttering I have achieved in the clinic and in my own studies that I want to share with you."

Many nonstutterers have become highly successful therapists for stutterers. Being a stutterer is not an essential qualification. An understanding of the nature of stuttering is vital both for the clinician and for the client.

I have no statistics concerning my success, such as the 95 percent rate claimed by Martin Schwartz or the 40 percent rate of George Shames, as he reported at a recent workshop in Modesto, California. My best guess is something like 75 percent, but percentage is elusive.

> We state confidently that, as a stutterer, you do not need to surrender helplessly to your speech difficulty because you can change the way you talk. You can learn to communicate with ease rather than with effort. There is no quick and easy way to tackle the problem, but, with the right approach, self-therapy can be effective. . . . Even with competent guidance, authorities would agree that stuttering therapy is largely a do-it-yourself project anyway. (Speech Foundation of America, No. 12, *Self-Therapy for the Stutterer*, 4th ed., p. 15–16.)

This book is a summation of my clinical experience and a review of the literature. I invite you to read, to ponder, and to apply the suggestions which are applicable to your case. You will need to select the sections which are personally useful. I am interested in your reactions to aid me in possible revisions.

# CONTENTS

# STUTTERING SELF-HELP
# FOR ADULTS

# Part I
# BACKGROUND INFORMATION

# REVIEW OF THE LITERATURE

ANTHONY GALLI

No speech pathology has caused more speculation, controversy, or conflicting research results than stuttering. Experts argue its definition, theory of causation, dynamics, measurement, and clinical management.

Stuttering has no widely accepted definition. Most dictionaries define stuttering as *hesitating or stumbling in uttering words*. Speech pathology experts describe stuttering variously. In one context, Wendell Johnson (1956) said, "stuttering is an *anticipatory apprehensive, hypertonic, avoidance reaction*" (p. 32). In other words, "stuttering is what a speaker does when he:

(1) expects stuttering to occur,
(2) dreads it,
(3) becomes tense in anticipation of it, and
(4) then even tries to avoid doing it."

According to Van Riper (1963) "Stuttering is

(1) when the flow of speech is broken by
    (a) hesitations,
    (b) stoppages,
    (c) repetitions, and/or
    (d) prolongations of the speech sounds.
(2) fluency is interrupted by
    (a) contortions,
    (b) tremors or
    (c) abnormalities of phonation and respiration.

(3) interruption of frequency as to
    (a) attract attention,
    (b) interfere with communication and
    (c) produce maladjustment.

5

(4) speech behavior that has been
    (a) labeled by others and
    (b) accepted by its possessor

as stuttering" (p. 306).

An estimated 1 percent of the population stutters, more men than women. The literature reveals a gender ratio of anywhere from 2:1, extending to a high of 9:1. The ratio of male to female stutterers appears to increase from childhood to adolescence (Milisen, 1957).

In appraising the differential gender ratio in stuttering, Schuell (1946, 1947) emphasized the following:

(1) Although the male child
    (a) is in many ways physiologically . . . more vulnerable

and

    (b) matures more slowly than the female child,
(2) he is . . .
    (a) subject to heavier demands for achievement . . .
    (b) receives inconsistent management, and
    (c) encounters more conflict with parental authority

than does the female. Schuell hypothesized that the gender differences in stuttering could be accounted for largely in terms of the differential treatment accorded boys and girls. By virtue of their experiences with inconsistencies in management and a general pattern of heavier demands, boys develop a more basic insecurity than do girls. This insecurity and anxiety become infused in their speech through both direct and indirect means.

Other experts define stuttering as *disruption in the fluency of verbal expression,* characterized by involuntary, audible or silent repetitions or prolongations in the utterance of short speech elements, such as sounds, syllables, and words of one syllable.

These disruptions

(1) usually

    (a) occur frequently or
    (b) are marked in character and
    (c) are not readily controllable.

(2) sometimes are accompanied by activities involving
   (a) the speech apparatus,
   (b) related or unrelated body structures, or
   (c) stereotyped speech utterances. (These activities appear to be speech-related struggle.)
(3) frequently are indications or reports of the presence of an emotional state ranging from
   (a) a general "excitement" or "tension"
   (b) to more specific negative emotions, i.e.,
      (i) fear,
      (ii) embarrassment,
      (iii) irritation.

The immediate source of stuttering is some incoordination expressed in the peripheral speech mechanism. The ultimate cause is presently unknown and may be complex or compound (Wingate, 1964, p. 498).

A quantitatively precise definition of stuttering is difficult. Perhaps stuttering is best characterized as *a cluster of particular speech behaviors, feelings, beliefs, self-concepts, and social interactions.* Each component may vary from person to person. In each person, the components can influence each other to generate a complicated problem involving disruptions of speech and the associated reactions. The emotional and social problems must be handled as well as the disordered speech.

## THE FOUR TRACKS OF STUTTERING

Van Riper (1982) believes that stuttering develops fairly consistently according to one of four major sequences or "tracks."

## Track I

Track I stutterers repeat syllables. (Single syllable words are repeated whole.) Initially, these syllabic repetitions are:

(1) *frequent*
(2) *multiple* —averaging about three per word, rarely exceeding five per word.
(3) *effortless* —no signs of awareness by the stutterer.
(4) *clustered*, followed by considerable normal fluency, thereby consti-

tuting only a small but very noticeable fraction of the total speech output. Additionally, these repetitions are spoken

(5) at the *same tempo* as the normally spoken syllables
(6) most frequently on the *first word after a pause or on the most meaningful word* of the sentence.

As the disorder develops, however, the pattern changes. The tempo of the disfluent syllables often increases. The repeated syllables become irregular. Then, first the range of the repetition increases and then the average number of repetitions.

Occasionally, prolonged "voiced continuant sounds" indicates that the stutter has developed even further. As the disorder continues to grow, the prolonged sounds move forward from the final repeated syllable of a series to the initial syllable. Very soon, prolonged sounds tend to dominate.

Next, surges of tension appear with obvious signs of struggle. The stutterer seeks to interrupt his closures and fixations. Facial contortions, jaw jerks, and comovements of the limbs are seen in various combinations. Much of this behavior almost appears random and unstereotyped. The tension, first located in the lips or jaws, overflows to adjacent structures. The stutterer is now highly aware of his difficulty, greatly frustrated by it, and doing his utmost to interrupt it so that he can communicate.

## Track II

One of the marked differences between Track I and Track II is that the fluency disruptions observed in Track II begin much earlier in speech development. Most, though not all, of Track II stutterers show retarded speech development and do not use phrases or sentences until they are three to six years of age. Distinctively, Track II stuttering begins right when connected speech does.

Early Track II behavior differs from that of Track I. In Track II, the initial syllabic repetitions are hurried and irregular, mostly one-syllable words. Later, Track II has more:

(1) silent gaps
(2) hesitations
(3) stumbling
(4) abortive beginnings
(5) revisions
(6) interjections

(7) back-ups
(8) retrials
(9) changes in direction.

than does Track I. Before they speak, Track II stutterers often hold their breath and then blurt. They seem to be searching for words. Articulation errors are prevalent.

Track II stutterers seem relatively frustration free. Their tolerance of disfluency seems very great, perhaps because so many of them have never known what it feels like to talk without stuttering. Moreover, awareness, fear, struggle, and avoidance develop more slowly than in Track I. This track also differs from Track I because prolonged sounds and fixations are rare. Track II stutterers repeat long strings of syllables or words, often very swiftly and compulsively, but they rarely hold a sound or articulatory posture during the early development of the disorder.

They also have fewer complete blockings of the airway at the lips, palate, or in the larynx in the later stages of development than do other stutterers.

## Track III

Track III stutterers speak quite fluently for several years. Since the age of onset is usually later than in Track II, Track III stutterers have experience with fluency. In Track III, the disorder starts very suddenly, beginning with an apparent inability to speak or to continue speaking. Track III stuttering can be engendered by shock—frightening experiences or sudden changes in environment. The stuttering is at first confined to the beginning of an utterance after a pause. Once the sentence or phrase begins, only a new utterance brings further difficulty. The basic initial behavior is fixation and not oscillation; tonic, not clonic. The first articulatory posture is held and prolonged. Tension and struggle accompany the stuttering almost from the beginning. The closure is primarily at the larynx. Breathing abnormalities now first occur and often become stereotyped rituals of attack. Overflow tension creates facial contortions and associated limb movements. Track III stutterers develop awareness and frustration almost immediately. Struggling and forcing also appear very soon. Tremors appear in the tensed muscles.

## Track IV

The onset of Track IV disorders is usually later than is the onset for other tracks. As in Track III, stuttering begins suddenly after several years of fluency. The initial behavior, however, is different. From the first, it seems highly stereotyped, almost deliberate and contrived. The stutterer seems very aware of the disorder from the first. He is even more aware of its impact on the listener, whom he watches carefully. In some of these stutterers, first comes repetitions of whole words or phrases rather than syllables; the repetitions soon change to include the latter. The initial word or phrase is repeated many more times than is usual in normal nonfluency. The inflection and intonation patterns may be demanding or insisting. The lengthy repetition of words already spoken normally is a continuously characteristic feature of Track IV stutterers. Even in the advanced stages, these stutterers sometimes say a word or phrase correctly, then stop and repeat it with pronounced dysfluency. Apparently, they return to the utterance only to stutter upon it.

Some stutterers who do not repeat, nevertheless, seem to belong in Track IV. First are gaps and pauses with stereotyped postures and activities, i.e., sobbing, grunting, biting, or tongue or lip protrusions. The jaws may be wide open with the sound of retching. Whimpering sounds with tremulous movements of the lower lip may fill the pauses.

One of the major distinguishing characteristics of Track IV is that the behavior changes very little over time. The frequency of stutterings may increase, but the basic patterns seem very stable. Few avoidance tricks are effective; disguise and masking behaviors are conspicuous by their absence and interrupter behaviors by their rarity. One can sense the controlling, punishing, and exploitative urges behind the stuttering behavior. These stutterers suffer less than do their listeners.

## THE PHASES OF STUTTERING

According to Bloodstein (1960), dysfluency may develop in various sequences.

## Phase I

Phase I dysfluency often occurs in preschool children who, fortunately, are usually too young to show concern or even awareness of dysfluency.

Phase I stuttering consists of episodic, repetitious dysfluency which occurs at the beginning of a sentence on small parts of speech and in situations of communication pressure.

## Phase II

Even though the primary school-aged, Phase II stutterer is old enough to see himself as a stutterer, he may show little or no concern. Major parts of speech are chronically dysfluent, and dysfluency increases during excitement or rapid speech.

## Phase III

Phase III dysfluency occurs most often in late childhood and in early adolescence; the stutterers still do not exhibit embarrassment. Although he begins to use sound substitutions, he does not avoid speech situations. Phase III stuttering is specific to situations and to certain sounds and words.

## Phase IV

Phase IV dysfluency, coming typically in later adolescence and adulthood, is the first phase to exhibit embarrassment and is marked by fearful anticipation of words, sounds, and speech situations. The Phase IV stutterer employs many word substitutions and begins to avoid speech.

## Causes of Stuttering

As with other communication disorders, classification of the numerous theories of causation of stuttering is based on inheritance, development, conditioning, and learning. These categories may overlap, and a specific theory may fit into more than one category. Stuttering may also be explained in terms of psychological or personality factors either in the stutterer himself or in his background. Even those theorists who believe in the importance of organic factors will frequently include psychological factors in their formulations of the etiology of stuttering.

A number of theories are relevant to the etiology of stuttering:

(1) **Anticipatory or struggle behavior** — The stutterer causes interference with his speech because he believes that speech is difficult or that he will fail. Three primary subtheories differ in etiology:

(a) *Communication failure theory* — Stuttering begins as a response to tension and fragmentation in speech brought about by continued and/or severe failures in communication under pressure.

(b) *Diagnosogenic theory* — Stuttering is caused by the misdiagnosis of normal dysfluencies in a child's speech, beginning the stuttering not, as it were, in the child's mouth but in the listener's ear.

(c) *Primary stuttering theory* — Stuttering emerges from a child's own normal hesitations and repetitions, occurring first without effort or awareness by the child. The stuttering develops when the child learns to anticipate, avoid, and fear speech situations because of listener reactions (Johnson, 1942).

(2) **Breakdown theory** — An individual possesses a constitutional predisposition toward stuttering which is precipitated by psychosocial or environmental stress. The precise nature of the predisposing factors and the extent to which heredity is an influence varies among the three primary subtheories:

(a) *Cerebral dominance and handedness* — One cerebral hemisphere is dominant for both speech and motor activities. A change in handedness presumably causes a disruption in the smooth flow of nerve impulses to the speech musculature, resulting in stuttering.

(b) *Symptomatic or biochemical* — Stuttering is a visible, outer symptom of an inner condition brought about by illness, by emotional or environmental stress, or by a biochemical imbalance.

(c) *Organic predisposition* — Stutterers have organic predispositions to motor and sensory perseveration, which manifests itself in the stuttering act (West, 1958).

(3) **Approach-avoidance theory** — Stuttering is caused by conflict between opposing drives to speak and to refrain from speaking. The stuttering block is the involuntary outcome of another learned approach — avoidance drives — and not itself a learned behavior (Sheehan, 1953).

(4) *Operant behavior theory* — Speech is a behavior under the operant control of positive and negative reinforcements; thus, stuttering has no single cause and is maintained by a complex schedule of reinforcements (Shames, 1963).

In summary, numerous theories posit an active agent within the child which causes stuttering. Such an agent may be constitutional or psychodynamic. Constitutionally, the specific agent may lie within the cortical activity affecting the speech areas; it may involve complex feedback circuits; or it may even involve an auditory feedback disturbance. Psychodynamically, the interruption in neural flow may be triggered by a primary anxiety. According to these theories, stuttering grows out of what the individual is. They essentially say, "He is this kind of person; therefore, he stutters."

On the other hand, some theories seek this active agent outside the child: in the listener, in the immediate environment, or in the culture itself. Other theories attempt to combine these and other possibilities in the active agent category, such as certain attitudes within the child plus an environmental factor such as social pressure.

Regarding the organic basis of stuttering, Eisenson (1958) hypothesized two opposing views:

(1) the original condition may cease to operate, or, conversely,
(2) the condition may continue into adulthood.

West (1958) believed that the cause of original repetitions disappear at puberty. Karlin (1947) believed that the condition ceases with completed myelinization. Glauber (1958) proposed that the alteration in ego structure may ultimately affect certain motor centers innervating the speech mechanism.

Therapy techniques tend to be geared to specific theoretical constructs. The ideas of Johnson (1967) for therapy showed his conviction that the listener's evaluation and the stutterer's resultant assumptions play a key role in the initiation of stuttering. Bloodstein (1961) suggested differential treatment for the four phases of development. He concentrated on therapy for stuttering as an anticipatory struggle reaction. Van Riper (1963) proposed treatment designed for his multiple origin perspective. Shoemaker (1967) designed therapeutic procedures dealing with learning theory concepts of stuttering. Sheehan (1958) uses combination of speech therapy and psychotherapy to gain understanding of feelings, relationships, and defenses. Sheehan's approach seeks to reduce avoidance by attacking word and situational fears. Those who see the stutterer as a neurotic or as one with a maldeveloped ego concentrate on psychotherapy to restructure the total personality (Cobb, 1943; Coriat, 1943).

Ritzman (1941) discussed as the essential causes of stuttering: parental coercion or lack of parental acceptance of the child, leading to repressed self-assertion in the child. Glasner (1949) reported that the majority of the stuttering children, although "not highly neurotic," were what are commonly referred to as "sensitive children" whose parents were over-protective, overanxious, and perfectionistic. Johnson (1944) has described parents of stutterers as likely to be perfectionists and inclined to have high standards for their children in cleanliness, table manners, toilet habits, and obedience as well as in speech proficiency.

In her study of stuttering children, Despert (1943) described the mothers as being generally domineering and overanxious, strict disciplinarians who manifested "maternal neurotic attitudes" towards oral activities, particularly in "the early eating-speaking situations."

Morgenstern (1956) found a significantly greater number of years between stutterers and their nearest siblings than between nonstutterers and their nearest siblings. He believed that widely-spaced children may receive more correction of their speech, leading to anxiety and self-consciousness about speech.

Duncan (1919) obtained questionnaire responses from stutterers which indicated that the stutterers felt their parents lacked real affection, did not understand them, underestimated their maturity, and were disappointed in them. Shultz (1947) also reported stutterers as indicating that they felt a lack of affection and that they frequently described their parents as dominating or irritating. Barbara (1946) found that the frequency of stutterers among psychotics was markedly lower than that reported in the general population. He stressed, however, that in every stuttering psychotic studied, either one or both parents were described as nervous, demanding, temperamental, rigid, and lacking in understanding. The family environment of these subjects was reported as being characterized by a lack of warmth and affection.

The literature reviewed contains what are essentially observational reports as well as experimental studies having adequate controls. Nonetheless, the authorities agree to a fairly impressive degree that the immediate environmental background of stutterers generally is emotionally unsatisfactory or conducive to stress and maladjustment.

## SPONTANEOUS RECOVERY

Researchers of stuttering behavior have performed intensive retrospective surveys. These studies generally report three categories: no recovery (students still stuttering), spontaneous recovery (recovery without therapy), and therapeutic recovery (recovery with therapy.) In the 1960s and 1970s, several surveys of incoming university students—young adults— probed stuttering history, and since the 1930s, surveys have also been made of children of various ages.

Probably the most extensive, and certainly the most widely-cited, cross-sectional studies of university students concerning the spontaneous recovery from stuttering are those of Sheehan and Martyn (1966, 1970) and Martyn and Sheehan (1968). These investigators conducted speech surveys of 5,138 new students entering the University of California. By means of speech samples, questionnaires, and personal interviews, the researchers identified 147 active or recovered stutterers. Of these 147 students, 31 (about 20%) were considered to be active stutterers. The remaining sample, 116 students (about 80%), reported stuttering previously. This study's most widely cited finding is that almost the entire 80 percent of young adults who report ever having stuttered also report that they recovered from their stuttering without intensive, formal treatment before entering college; only a neglible number reported recovery with therapy. Essentially:

| | |
|---|---|
| no recovery: | 20% |
| spontaneous recovery: | 80% |
| therapeutic recovery: | 0% |

Cooper, Paris, and Wells (1974) essentially replicated the Sheehan and Martyn procedures with over 7000 incoming students at the University of Alabama, with significantly different results. These authors found that 82 percent of the students who reported stuttering also reported recovering from stuttering before entering college, with or without therapy. Of this 82 percent, however, 37.5 percent (30% of the total sample) reported having received speech therapy, leaving only 52 percent reporting spontaneous recovery, statistically, a very significant difference of almost 30 percent from the previous three studies by Sheehan and Martyn. Essentially:

| | |
|---|---|
| no recovery: | 18% |
| spontaneous recovery: | 30% |
| therapeutic recovery: | 52% |

Porfert and Rosenfield (1978) surveyed University of Massachusetts students, finding that approximately 62 percent of the students who reported stuttering also reported recovery before entering college (with or without therapy).

Essentially,

> no recovery:                     28%
> spontaneous recovery
> and therapeutic recovery:    62%

Patricia Johnson (1951) studied 23 former stutterers; all but one were college students between the ages of 17 and 31. By recalling former symptoms, her subjects indicated adequately once having stuttered. Most could not state a definite age of onset of stuttering, but each could recall having begun to stutter prior to a certain age, usually age eight. Twelve rated their former stuttering as mild, ten as average, and one as severe. They also recalled their feelings about stuttering; five said that they had been relatively indifferent to it. The other 18, however, reported having had various personal reactions, including annoyance, worry, embarrassment, shame, impatience, or inferiority. Some felt challenged or handicapped. The majority of subjects still referred to their past stuttering as a handicap or inferiority.

Most of the subjects also recalled reactions from peers, parents, or teachers. These "outside" reactions, especially from the latter two, appeared to Johnson to be "an active, not a passive influence, in the majority of instances . . . " and one which " . . . constituted a critical source in these persons' environment[s]" (Wingate, 1976, p. 96).

Parental reactions varied. Six persons indicated that their parents did not think the stuttering was particularly important. The other 17 reported, however, that their parents had been concerned about the stuttering. Behavioral science researchers generally agree that data based upon subject memory are so unreliable as to be of questionable value. Relying on subject memory for information about the onset or recovery of stuttering is particularly problematic because it is difficult to cross-validate such information.

Wingate (1964) obtained information from 50 recovered stutterers, 32 males and 18 females from 17 to 54 years old, with an average age of 34. All reported having stuttered for at least two years, most of them for five years or more. Although all of the subjects considered themselves to be "recovered," only half described their speech as that of a normally fluent individual. The other half said that they had residual tendencies to stutter, usually describing some minimal, transitory, easily controlled stuttering, possibly reappearing under particular stress. They added that these tendencies present no problem in communication or in their personal adjustment. They indicated that they were regarded as normal speakers by their friends and acquaintances, and that most people evidently were not aware that they might occasionally "really" stutter.

# POSSIBLE CAUSES OF STUTTERING

In the United States, more than a million persons stutter or have stuttered at any one time. You, as one of them, have found stuttering to be a baffling and sometimes maddening aspect of living. "Why should I have this affliction?" you ask. "Why can't I speak fluently?"

Professional speech therapists in all parts of the United States have been studying the problem of the nonfluent speaker. They have found data which will be of interest to you. General agreement is that stuttering is not physical in nature; there is nothing wrong with the functioning of the lungs, vocal cords, or muscles of articulation. The tongue, for example, works perfectly well for chewing food and for swallowing. Only when speech is involved does the tongue seem to "act up" or "get stuck." As long ago as 1894, Dr. Leopold Treitel, a German physician, called stuttering a nervous disorder. Today various terms are used, such as "semantic," "psychic," or "emotional," but they all add up to the conclusion that stuttering is the result of the attitude of the speaker toward the speaking situation.

Although many researchers and therapists believe that there are no significant physical differences between stutterers and nonstutterers, some national authorities, e.g., Charles Van Riper, include muscular incoordination of the articulator as an underlying cause of stuttering. The cause of this predisposing organicity is unknown but may be genetic. Using electromyographic techniques, researchers found evidence of abnormal functioning of the larynx, tongue, and breathing mechanism. Controversy remains regarding cause and effect: Does this mistiming cause stuttering? Or is the mistiming itself a result of tension during episodes of dysfluency? Both the stutterer and the clinician need to accept the possibility of an organic predisposition but realize that, if this is the case, they are powerless to erase this cause. At a slower rate of speech, this incoordination is diminished.

We know that there is no ready cure, no panacea for stuttering. Schools have been set up which guarantee cures in a few weeks, but, unfortunately, most of the participants have failed to receive permanent benefits. Over-coming your stuttering is likely to be a long and very gradual process. Most authorities agree that the adult stutterer will always stutter, at least at times. You may, however, learn to control the repetitions or hesitations so well that your nonfluency will be unobserved—except on "bad days."

Certain other data have been collected by the research departments of university speech clinics. There is a tendency for stuttering to run in families. The question remains, however, whether stuttering in inherited. More likely, the environment provided by such families affects various members of the family. A mother is more watchful of speech production in her young son if Uncle Jack or Cousin Bess is a stutterer. She is more inclined to interpret the normal hesitancies and sputterings of the young child as undesirable.

At one time there was a great deal of writing about the relationship of handedness and stuttering. Researchers felt that a lack of hand prefer-ence or a change from left- to right-handedness was the major cause of stuttering. Further research tended to disprove such a direct relationship but to conclude that a forced change of handedness might be one of the causal factors. Now parents are advised to allow the children to develop handedness on their own, without interference. Although it might be easier to be right-handed in our particular society, left-handedness should be accepted as a perfectly normal characteristic.

Some people believe that stuttering is caused by a traumatic situation in the early life of the individual. The stutterer may have been bitten by a dog, or witnessed the death of the father or experienced some other harrowing event. But when a complete case history is taken, the fact usually remains that the stuttering was apparent before the shocking experience. Nor is it likely that stuttering is "caught" by imitating someone in the immediate environment, such as a playmate or relative.

Thus far, we have stressed what stuttering is not, or what factors do not cause it. What, then *does* cause stuttering?

Innumerable theories exist about the genesis of the "affliction," as some of my stuttering patients have described their condition. Many factors probably combine to cause stuttering in any one individual. None of these factors, in itself, would be potent enough to cause a breakdown in speech, but the cumulative effect is disastrous. An under-standing of the "multiple causation" basis of stuttering is essential in setting up a program to rid oneself of it. Another way of saying the same thing is that an accumulation of environment pressures causes stuttering.

Most stutterers say that they have had trouble with their speech as long as they can remember. They may have become acutely aware of it when they were in the upper grades or in high school, but it actually started long before that. In many cases, the individuals have improved in terms of fluency and then taken a turn for the worse about the time they entered high school. Your speech irregularities may have started when you were four or five. For a time, you improved. Then, at adolescence, your speech became increasingly nonfluent.

A beginning point in overcoming your stuttering is "insight" into how and why it began. One authority in the field of speech correction, who was himself a severe stutterer, has stated that the completely happy child will not stutter. So the search begins to find those factors which made your childhood less satisfactory than it might have been. To undertake such an investigation, you must be nonsentimental about your home situation.

Then, too, how you as a child felt about the childhood environment is far more important than how it really was. This last fact partly explains why two children may be exposed to approximately the same environmental situation and react in entirely different ways. They feel differently about it. One stutters and the other doesn't. Or one may have additional pressures which the other one does not experience. No two children, even in the same family, have exactly the same environment. Age differs, even in cases of multiple births; gender may differ, as may physical attractiveness (or perceptions of). So we are not particularly interested in how you should have felt about the childhood environment— feeling has little logic. Nor are we interested, at least not at this point, in how you feel about it *now,* but—how did you feel about the environment at *that* time—at the time you were four, or seven, or fourteen?

None of the factors which we discuss here may apply to your case, but they may suggest areas about which you can think further. So often, patients say, "But I never thought about that. I had no idea there was any connection between that and the way I speak." But your speech is a reflection of you. You are a product of all the thoughts and feelings which you have ever had. Your current attitudes are outgrowths of many years of thinking about and reacting to your immediate surroundings. For all of us, that means our reactions and attitudes towards our family members. So now we are ready to examine more closely some of the factors which made your childhood less than ideal.

### 1. Were your parents divorced?

Divorce is very common today, yet children can still react to divorce as a direct blow to their security. The effect of divorce can be reflected in a child's speech patterns. If your parents were divorced, you may have said nothing about the break-up of the home, even though you probably felt it deeply. Perhaps, if you were silent, the wonder and doubt began to come through as a speech problem. Cause, guilt. If you were between the ages of three and five when your parents divorced, the odds of a resultant speech defect are increased. All aspects of relationship need to be re-examined. Was financial child support lacking, insufficient, or inconsistent? Was the parental post-divorce relationship otherwise strained? Was visitation a bone of contention?

### 2. If not, did the family atmosphere have an undercurrent of tension?

Tension which is not expressed directly can often have even more insidious effects than open argument. Your parents may never have quarreled openly in your presence. Consciously or subconsciously, you may have been aware of dissension. Or, if your parents were merely undemonstrative, you may have felt they lacked real companionship. You might have been afraid that at any time the tensions could explode, leaving you homeless. In many cases, stuttering adults have reported to me that they urged, or wanted to urge a parent—usually the mother—to "get out," to get a divorce.

Parents who consistently function well as a unit are the keystone to a secure family. Overcoming speech problems in children often begins with assisting the parents in solving their problems. As the parents become more relaxed and accepting of each other, they also become more accepting of the children as individuals, although dependent, units of the family. They no longer need to use the child as a pawn in a battle of the sexes, nor to use the child to supply sympathy and/or affection which should be supplied by each other.

### 3. Was there competition between/among the children?

Often the stuttering child is one who feels "second best" in an "affection competition," real or imagined, within the family. Suppose your family had two sons, you and a younger brother. Your younger brother seemed to be more athletic than you, more socially acceptable. He could read faster, he was better in mathematics, a better student all around.

Charles was a year older than his brother Bob. After Charles failed an early grade, the brothers were in the same class throughout grade school. Bob always got higher grades. Even though their parents never pointed out the difference in their achievements, the fact was all too apparent. In fact, once, in the fifth grade, a thoughtless teacher remarked, "If you'd try a little harder, you might catch up with your brother Bob." In high school, Bob was an outstanding athlete as well as an honor student and won a scholarship to an eastern college. Charles, admiring, never complaining, seemed never to begrudge Bob his honors, but he stuttered so badly that he could hardly say a complete sentence.

In many instances, however, parents do aggravate the situation by showing favoritism. One woman, Jane, told me that her father always took her sister's side in every situation. The mother, hoping family peace would return sooner if she refused to take sides, remained impartial. In many insidious ways, the father let Jane know that she was less attractive, less acceptable to him than her sister. Did Jane stutter? Yes, quite severely. She left home to find a new beginning in California.

#### 4. Did your parents set standards which were too high?

The high standards may have been in areas other than speech. Philip, for instance, was the son of a lawyer; his mother had been an English teacher before marriage. From his earliest school years, they insisted that Philip stand in the upper third of his class. "It isn't," they would say, "as if we expect you to be the highest." But Philip was only average in academic capacities. Try as hard as he might, he was able to get only a little above average, and sometimes not even that. Although his report card showed: "Satisfactory for this child," his parents were never satisfied. He loved his parents, and it made him unhappy to disappoint them. Every time the report cards came out, he felt a sense of guilt and shame. His stuttering was always worse at these times.

Some early studies showed that the mothers of stutterers, as a group, were tense, high-strung, perfectionistic individuals. One speech pathologist facetiously remarked, "If there were no mothers, there would be no stutterers." This pathologist had a point, but it was too narrow. Mothers, fathers, grandparents, even aunts, uncles, cousins, etc., who force their goals, realistic or unrealistic, onto children are the precipitating forces behind many stuttering cases.

### 5. Did your parents insist on running your life?

Louise was a nice-looking girl, healthy and athletic. She was fond of animals and the outdoors and wanted to work as a summer camp waitress. Her family thought that well-connected young ladies did not do such a thing. She would go to summer school to make up credits and then enter a girls' finishing school in the fall. This was only one in a series of situations in which Louise's wishes were subordinated to her family's goals for her. If she did not feel herself to be the black sheep of the family, at least she felt that she was the weak link in the chain of generations. Her fluency began to improve after college graduation when she established herself as an independent individual.

### 6. Were your parents overcontrolling?

Your parents may have been of the "children are to be seen and not heard" school. John developed apprehension in terms of speech. Not only was his nervous mother unable to stand loud noise, but his father worked at night. Therefore, the house had to be quiet for his father to sleep during the day. John was constantly cautioned to be quiet, not to talk so loud. Whenever John forgot and talked too loud—perhaps even at normal levels, he was punished. Once, his father shouted from the bedroom, "Mary, can't you make that kid keep his mouth shut?" Talking, at least the kind of talking John did, was considered bad. "Good boys are quiet and don't talk needlessly. They censor their speech."

Perhaps, you did not always say the right things (what child does?). Or you were not naturally a quiet child—and, seemingly, few are. But if your parents attempted to overcontrol these natural childish tendencies, possibly you began to hesitate to speak. You strained with a child's lack of precision for the too narrow range of acceptable speech. Naturally, you were often unsuccessful. This fear of speaking "incorrectly" became more pronounced, until others began to remark about your stuttering.

### 7. Were inconsistent standards or degrees of discipline used in your upbringing?

Were you allowed to do something by one parent and not by the other? If there was another adult relative in the home, did that person enforce different rules from those of your parents? At the age of three or four, perhaps you were confused about the limits of your activities. Even if you learned to play one parent against the other, you were not really happy about getting your way. You were always afraid of being found out and punished. In terms of your state of mind—and, indirectly, in terms of your speech—parents should consistently enforce a few rules rather than inconsistently enforcing many. Vascillating methods, degrees, or standards of discipline are worse than severity in developing a child's sense of security, which affects so many other aspects of development.

### 8. Were you neglected by your parents as they kept you at a physical or emotional distance or both?

A child needs to feel that some one, especially a parent, is interested in him or her. A child's feeling that no one is interested can cause severe psychological damage.

Martin's father was a traveling salesman, and Martin's mother wished to accompany him on his route. Martin's parents were overcome by traveling with a child, so Martin was left with his grandparents most of the time. As soon as he was old enough, his parents sent him to military school. The father lost all interest in his son. The parents divorced, and the father disappeared completely from Martin's life. The mother visited Martin once or twice a year and allowed Martin to spend part of the summer vacation with her and Martin's new stepfather. Throughout his school life, Martin's stuttering was a handicap to him, which he overcame when he graduated and assumed responsibility for his own professional and social activities.

### 9. Did your parents have considerable financial worries, creating insecurity?

You, as a young child, probably were not directly concerned with financial worries. However, tension over money problems will still have had an effect upon the home. As a sensitive individual, you may have imagined the situation to be even worse than it was. This apprehension could have been intensified if one or both of your parents were pessimistic about the prospects of future financial success for the family. Arguments over money may have been held in the presence, or at least within the hearing, of the children.

Ruth was very conscious of her family's lack of financial resources. Her earliest memories were concerned with her mother's constant fussing and fuming about what "we can't afford." She dressed Ruth neatly but in clothes inferior in quality to those of most of her classmates. Once she complained about wearing "that old brown dress," and her mother gave her a very severe lecture about trying to put on airs. After that, Ruth held her remarks, but her desires to have pretty clothes and trinkets like the other girls caused her great unhappiness. She began to withdraw from her social group and to speak with considerable hesitation. When her father got a better job, the money worries were relieved. Gradually, she began to regain her self-confidence. As she did so, her speech improved.

A situation similar to constant financial stress, creating uncertainty, is that of recurrent unemployment. Dale's father had quit school as a high school junior, drifting aimlessly until he met and married Dale's mother. Then he began to "settle down," but he was not trained for any occupation. He was also often very outspoken against his bosses. As a consequence, he was forced to take unskilled labor jobs which were not too much to his liking. By the time Dale was four years old, his father had worked at more than fifteen jobs. The family had also moved six times. Dale often asked his father, "Are you going to look for a job today?" Perhaps it is no surprise that Dale stuttered.

**10. Were either or both of your parents extremely overprotective?**

The effects of extreme overprotectiveness are almost invariably deleterious. An extremely overprotective parent hovers over children, shielding them from every danger, providing them with every comfort. Such a parent sacrifices completely for the family, having almost no interests outside the home. An only child, perhaps, suffers the most in this situation, receiving the full force of devotion.

Such a parent does not allow you to grow and develop as a normal individual, waiting on you to such an extent that you fail to learn to do things for yourself. You become "spoiled" and find it difficult to make satisfactory contacts with other children. At times, you lash out against this overprotection, then feel guilty because the parent's feelings are hurt. You love the parent but wish you would be allowed to live your own life.

This constant emotional hassle resulted in mixed feelings of liking and disliking. Later, overprotected as you were, making decisions for yourself became increasingly difficult. Even as an adult, perhaps, you cannot break the home ties and are still living with your parents.

A few years back, the press centered a great deal of attention on "Momism." Now recognized as a sexist term, Momism is treated with more understanding as the result of almost overpowering social forces on women's role modeling. The effects of Momism, whatever its causes, can be damaging to normal emotional development of children.

**11. Did your family or others make you aware of your speech problem, either jokingly or cruelly?**

Some authorities maintain that you began to stutter simply because someone told you that you stuttered. By calling attention to your "different" speech, people caused you to retain and carry along a pattern of speech that is perfectly normal during early phases of speech development. Although this explanation fails to take into consideration the numerous possible causes of stuttering, it does stress the importance of other people's attitudes toward your speech. Some persons in your environment, probably parents, were anxious about your speech and transmitted that anxiety to you. A grandparent or neighbor may have been the person who made you conscious that your speech was unacceptable.

In addition to making you conscious that your speech is nonfluent, listeners simply do not know what to do with a stutterer. The most perplexed and frustrated listener is the one who feels he or she is in a position of authority and therefore should do *something* to indicate disapproval of this unacceptable behavior. This self-imposed or actual authority figure may have felt that to ignore the problem was dishonest, unhelpful, or both. Unwittingly, this well-intentioned "help" may have only made matters worse. Examples are:

> "Slow down;" (you would if you could)
> "Stop and take a deep breath;" (it doesn't help)

"Think before you speak;" (as if you weren't, implying that stuttering is a "thoughtless" activity that could be controlled if only one's mind were put to it with proper concentration) and similar admonitions only intensified the environmental pressures.

Members of the family or others making fun of the stuttering is especially damaging to the ego.

You really would not stutter if you could help it. For others to call attention to the speech in any way, as well meaning as they may be, only makes the situation worse.

---

As an adult stutterer, you may be comforted to realize that you were not responsible for the beginnings of your stuttering. In the primary stage of your speech problem, you were unaware that you were producing speech that differed from that of your playmates. Gradually, however, you became increasingly aware that something was wrong. If the situation had been handled properly at that time, your stuttering might have been "cured." But, unfortunately, that was not so. The attitudes persisted that:

1. You would grow out of it;
2. You could speak correctly if you wanted to; and/or
3. You were enjoying the attention you received from stuttering.

As the years passed, you moved on to the second stage of stuttering. You were fully aware of your speech trouble; you avoided speech situations whenever possible. Many times you said, "I don't know" rather than make an effort to answer substantively. In high school, you began to withdraw from social groups and to refuse to recite in class. You had almost no dates because you were afraid to ask a girl out, or to accept a date. And you wouldn't use the telephone. Throughout college, social situations became increasingly difficult. You turned to nonverbal activities, such as reading or listening to music, for recreation.

As an adult, you still stutter, although probably not as severely as in your teens. Stuttering remains a major communication problem, however, especially on bad days.

Finding a job is possibly difficult because oral interviews are troublesome. You might stick with an unpleasant job rather than seek one which could require speaking to the public. You refuse to use the telephone except in emergencies.

At this point, stuttering is more than a communication problem; it is really interfering with your whole life, your development as a human being—both professionally and socially. Finally, you have come to the point where you feel you must do something to overcome this stumbling block.

# Part II
# 13 STEPS TOWARD
# OVERCOMING STUTTERING

---

Before you study and practice through *The 13 Steps Toward Overcoming Stuttering,* I recommend that you read my adaptation of Anthony Galli's *Review of the Literature.* The discussions of the definitions of stuttering, possible causes, and spontaneous recovery are enlightening. The information is also important to your understanding of the "enemy," stuttering. The more you know about your condition, the more likely you will be successful in your battle to improve fluency. You may prefer to start the steps toward fluency and read Galli's research findings as your schedule permits.

# Step 1

# FACING UP TO THE PROBLEM

### Step Ia: Admitting That There Is a Problem in Fluency

*Do you admit — to yourself and to your listeners — that you have a speech problem? Can you say, "I am a stutterer?"*

This simple statement is basic to getting started on a program for the improvement of your fluency. Any denial on your part sabotages the program from the beginning.

Additionally, you must learn to talk about your disfluency to others. With whom to start your campaign for exposure of your "secret" is a decision you must make on your own. In clinical programs, the first listener would be a well trained and sympathetic speech therapist. In a self-help program, possible first listeners include relatives or close friends. Some stutterers have actually found it easier to begin with strangers whom they do not expect to see again.

Eventually, however, the information must come "home" through you to people in your immediate inner circle. Slowly, you then begin to spread the information, possibly among people you trust. Even if those of your original inner circle learn of the stuttering indirectly, you must ultimately learn to be able to face the problem with new people of potential importance to you. Otherwise, your stutter will continue to hamper you. You will continue to fear its exposure.

In a self-help program, sharing the acknowledgement of your stuttering has another purpose. You will need someone to help you observe and analyze your stuttering pattern in the identification process of Step 4.

Numerous cases have been reported in the literature of stutterers who have never mentioned their speech problem to their spouses. Obviously, the spouse is aware of the abnormalities in the speech of the marriage partner, but the couple has never discussed it.

In some cases, adults undertake programs of speech therapy "on the sly" and have requested that their relatives, including spouses, children, parents, and siblings not be informed. These adults have been fearful of lack of improvement and prefer that persons in their inner circle be

31

unaware of their attempt to correct the problem. Such secrecy is not necessarily bad in the early stages of therapy, but the goal is to overcome the reluctance to reveal the truth as soon as possible. When both the speaker (stutterer) and the listener can talk openly about the speech problem, the lines of oral communication are greatly extended.

In a recent workshop of the local chapter of the National Stuttering Project (NSP) one participant explained his method of handling the situation: He worked in an office, and as new customers came in, he would tell them immediately that he might be hesitant in his speech. He found that this information made further oral communication much easier. Rarely, in his experience, did anyone react adversely. The possibility of some disfluencies was out in the open, and the discussants were much less tense in talking about the business at hand.

Stutterers who are called upon to speak before groups often find it preferable to mention their speech problem. The air is cleared immediately when the stutterer announces, "I may have some difficulty with my speech. I am working on my problem, but it sometimes still pops up."

In sum, you are admitting both to yourself and to the listener that you are not trying to hide the problem. Frequently, this first step is not easy to accomplish. One lady in her 60's at the NSP workshop stated that she still is unwilling to take this first step toward improved fluency. We can fairly safely assume that she would have been more successful in her efforts to overcome her stuttering if she had been able to admit and communicate her problem forty or fifty years ago. At that time, too, it probably would have been easier for her to "expose" her problem. Unfortunately, the idea probably wasn't presented to her then; if so, evidently not forcefully enough.

In a 1988 movie, "Clean and Sober," the main character (played by Michael Keaton) voluntarily checks into a private clinic specializing in problems of drug addiction and alcoholism. In group sessions, the counselor asks the participants if they are addicted or if they are alcoholics or both. Unless they answer in the affirmative, they are asked to drop out of the program. *First step:* ADMIT THE PROBLEM.

Do what you can to make your own road toward improved fluency as short as possible. Start right now on the right foot by wasting no time in admitting the problem to yourself. Now, think of one other person you can tell. Right now DO IT.

Remember always that you are not alone. At least 1 percent of the population has a similar problem. In this group a significant number have become famous. Jock Carlisle has compiled the following list.

> The Clan of the Tangled Tongue includes the prophet Moses and the philosophers Demosthenes and Aristotle. Emperors and kings (Emperor Claudius of Rome, and kings Charles I and George VI of England) and statesmen (Thomas Jefferson, Winston Churchill, and Aneuran Bevan) stuttered, and some well-known scientists (Isaac Newton, Erasmus Darwin, and Charles Darwin) and authors (Virgil, Aesop, Charles Lamb, Nevil Shute, Arnold Bennett, and Somerset Maugham) had trouble with their speech. Some public figures, film stars, television personalities, and musicians (Lorne Green, Eric Roberts, Marilyn Monroe, Gary Moore, Jack Paar, Annie Glenn, and Mel Tillis) managed to cope in public in spite of their blocks and hesitations, and many professors of speech pathology, psychiatrists, and speech therapists have been troubled by tangled tongues, particularly the eminent Wendell Johnson, Charles Van Riper, Joseph Sheehan, Hugo Gregory, and Einer Boberg.
>
> The list is endless. All these people rose to prominence by great effort and courage in spite of their stuttering (1985, p. 15).

## Step 1b: *Motivation and Commitment*

*Do you have adequate motivation to persist in a program of remediation? Are you determined to give priority to such a program in terms of time and effort?*

During the first interview with an adult stutterer who is applying for speech therapy we always ask, in one way or another, "Why are you asking for help with your stuttering problems?"

Typical replies include the following:

1. My boss tells me I can't be promoted unless I talk better.

2. My parents have been after me for twenty years to do something about my speech.

3. My son is beginning to talk, and I don't want him to stutter.

4. I had therapy in school, but I didn't carry out the clinician's instructions. Now I've decided to try again.

5. I just met a person who interests me, and I don't want to look stupid.

6. I think my stuttering has held me back socially and professionally. I'm tired of this albatross around my neck.

And so it goes. Stutterers have different reasons for entering therapy. These reasons are good, but a clinician must decide whether they are adequate for success. Even in a joint venture between clinician and student, often the two are trying to change fluency patterns which have persisted for ten, fifteen, or even thirty years. In most cases, the longer the stuttering problem has existed, the more difficult it is to modify these melodic patterns. If the clinician discovers that the stutterer is being pushed into therapy by significant others, such as parent, love interest, or employer, the clinician may suggest that the stutterer postpone therapy.

Some speech pathologists, such as Charles Van Riper, believe that part of the clinician's professional responsibility is to build and maintain motivation. Motivation is integral to the therapy process. In times of discouragement, when improvement is minimal or even nonexistant, such a clinician will shift emphasis to motivational factors until the crisis or plateau has passed.

In self-help programs, however, no clinician is available. All motivation must come from within the stutterer. Unless you have considerable determination, the likelihood of abandoning the program is extremely high.

Realistically, then, you must evaluate honestly whether you are the one who demands changes in your speech. To enter a therapy program, with or without actual clinical sessions, in a half-hearted manner is to court failure.

As mentioned earlier in this book, you know that most stutterers have overcome their speech problems, with or without clinical sessions, by adulthood. When you realize that over 75 percent of childhood stutterers have only occasional disfluent periods, then your attitude may well be, "If all these people have overcome stuttering, then I can certainly join this multitude of ex-stutterers."

**Step 1c:** *Responsibility for Problem—Perseverance and Progress*

*Whose fault is it that you stutter? Who's responsible for getting rid of it? What if it all just seems too much? To whom can you turn if you just don't seem to be making any progress?*

As, you can tell, responsibility is closely related to motivation. You must recognize that stuttering and its remission are your problem. You are not responsible for creating the factors that caused you to stutter in the first place, but you are responsible that you continue to stutter because only you can change it. This does not mean that stuttering is your fault, simply that you are doing it. You are the stutterer. Only you can stop it. Only you have the authority to cause change within yourself.

Certainly, others can provide support, but you must accept primary responsibility for sustaining the necessary effort to bring significant progress in fluency. All the support in the world can't bring about the change if you are not committed to it.

Considerable clinical experience has made me aware of gaps between what stutterers say and what they basically believe. Too often students give the impression that they will make an all-out commitment to gain adequate fluency. Perhaps they even verbalize this apparent commitment. Yet many of these students fail to carry through on a day-to-day basis. I have observed this failure in children, especially teenagers, and even in some adults.

I have discovered what I believe is often the underlying attitude— possibly even a subconscious one—which prevents progress in these cases. The real attitude of the student is:

> *Here I am, a stutterer. You are the expert. So cure me. Solve my problem for me.*

Such an attitude will defeat any effort to make significant progress in changing stuttering patterns. The major effort—especially in a self-help approach to therapy—is yours.

Joseph Sheehan, who was a nationally known psychologist and speech pathologist at the University of California, Los Angeles, has written:

> *Learning the Language of Responsibility.* Your stuttering is not something that happens to you, but something that you do. See if you can observe and describe your stuttering in language that recognizes that you have a part in it, that it is your own behavior. You are doing the doing. You have responsibility and you have a choice.

You must say to yourself,

> *I am the will behind this behavior. I can control it. My will is now allowing this behavior to happen. I can change my will and change this behavior. My will is stronger than the forces which are causing this behavior. My will can outlast those forces and beat them. This is true no matter how long it takes, how tired or discouraged I get. I will wait, and recharge and get back in the fight. I may get down, but never out.*

Lloyd Hulit, a stutterer and Professor of Speech Pathology at Illinois State University in Normal, Illinois, states, "If you want flency enough that you are willing to make speech a high priority in your life, you have an excellent chance for realizing your potential" (1985).

In his case, he made such a decision when he entered high school. He looked for every opportunity to test himself—to speak and to act. In college he majored in public speaking, theatre, and mass communications. The most important factor in his success was determination to be fluent. He had to make the necessary effort, to go out and find the roughest challenges, and to make the adjustments which were necessary for a better performance the next time.

# Step 2

# IDENTIFYING THE SYMPTOMS

*Are you capable of studying your pattern of stuttering so that you are fully aware of what you do in speaking that marks you as a stutterer?*

This is extremely tricky for a couple of reasons. First of all, how can you tell? You don't know until you have tried, and even then, how do you judge your attempt? Second of all, several demanding skills are required to complete this step successfully:

high degrees of: perception<br>
objectivity

Step 2 is identifying the specifics of your stutter. Definitions of stuttering include descriptions of the symptoms of the condition. These symptoms can be divided into three subgroups:

1) the interruptors of the flow of speech
    a) repetitions
    b) prolongations
    c) blockings
2) secondary physical results of stuttering
    a) irregular breathing
    b) eye blinks
    c) head turning
    d) lip pressing
    e) irrelevant movement of extremities
        i) fingers
        ii) hands
        iii) feet
3) negative emotions
    a) frustration
    b) shame
    c) anger.

You need a sample of your stuttered speech. The sample should not be memorized or even practiced but as spontaneous as possible to simulate natural speech. The only advance preparation should be to think of topics about which you could speak for at least 150 words.

Monitoring your own speech while you are creating it is almost impossible, even with a mirror to reflect the physical characteristics to you. The sample should also be observed or at least listened to more than once to check the recorded characteristics. Repeating a spontaneous speech would be difficult. If you do more than one run-through, repeating exactly what you said before, the stuttering pattern will not be exactly the same. Even another person might have trouble listening, watching, and accurately noting and recording all the characteristics simultaneously with only one run-through. You could "talk to the air," but it would be more natural if you have a conversation with the friend.

If you have recorded your sample, however, you can replay a recording as many times as needed to get an accurate count of repetitions, prolongations, and distractions. Ideally, your stuttering sample should be videotaped. That way, even the visual distractions can be replayed; slow speed can be used for greater detail. Since most of us do not have access to videotaping, the second best sample is an audio tape. The difficulty with an audio tape is that since your physical distraction will not show up, you only get one chance to record them. Someone other than the speaker can observe and record more accurately, so he or she must do this as you are recording.

If you made a recording in a room by yourself with no listener involved, your speech will probably not be typical but uncharacteristically fluent. A more typical sample is possible if you are speaking spontaneously to another person in a natural situation.

If you can, get one person to be the listener and one to be the recorder. This makes it easier on everyone. The sample will be more natural. You usually do not speak to someone who is writing, much less noting how you are speaking. The listener can just listen, maybe commenting afterwards on how distracting the different characteristics were for the listener. A video tape can make a more accurate recording of the visual distractions.

Here is where some of those people to whom you have acknowledged your stuttering can come in handy. Go back to those people from Step 2 and ask one or two to help you with your stuttering by sitting in as listener or recorder.

Another idea is to turn on the tape recorder as you make a telephone call. Most stutterers have considerable difficulty in this speaking situation. You automatically have a listener on the other end of the line (even though they can't comment on the visual distractions) so you only need an observer to record the visual distractions.

To arrive at the most natural situation, the taping should be done with your permission but not with your knowledge that it is being done at that particular moment. You may be slightly self-conscious knowing that the taping could be being done at any moment (with obvious exceptions), but you may become so involved in some conversation that you will forget the possibility.

Perhaps you cannot make a recording of which you are unaware, because of circumstances, preference, or inability to forget the possibility. The situation is then slightly unnatural since you know that you are being recorded and watched. Still try to make the situation as natural and low-key as possible, maybe going outdoors or to a cafeteria. You need someplace relatively quiet so that the stuttering can be clearly recorded. Possibly the recorder could wear a lapel microphone. The recorder should sit so that he or she can see the face of the stutterer but as much out of sight of the stutterer as possible. If a clinical setting is the only one available due to weather, noise, crowding, or whatever, a slight advantage may be had if the recorder can sit on the other side of a one-way mirror.

The process of identification of stuttering symptoms is important so that you realize what you do when you stutter. Step 2 is also a prerequisite to Step 3, where you administer to yourself the Stuttering Severity Inventory (SSI). You need to spend enough time on Step 2 to feel confident in your ability to recognize and count single incidents of stuttering behavior, including *involuntary:*

1) repetitions
   a) single sounds
   b) syllables (other than one-syllable words)
   c) phrases (other than for emphasis or rephrasing)
2) prolongations
   a) silent (blocks)
   b) vocalized
3) distractions
   a) facial
   b) head and neck
   c) extremities
   d) body

One aspect of your speech which does not show up directly on the SSI from Step 3 is the amount of fluent speech which you usually have. In other words, what proportion of your speech is stuttered and what proportion fluent? Under what circumstances is the stuttering more likely to occur? Under these circumstances, does it always occur? If not, how often? On "good days," possibly over 80 percent of your speech may be fluent. Only in rare cases does a stutterer have disfluencies all the time.

Most stutterers are pleasantly surprised to discover just how fluent they really are. The identification phase of therapy helps you to be realistic about the severity of your problem. Perhaps it is much less severe than you believe, perhaps because others have led you to so believe. Obviously, you do stutter to some degree or you wouldn't be interested in a program of remediation. Appendix I examines a publication about advice which former stutterers give. The second most frequent bit of advice is:

"You, as a stutterer, must study your speech patterns in order to become aware of the differences between stuttered and fluent speech."

I would add to this that you must become aware of the specific differences between *your* stuttered and fluent speech.

Step 3

# MEASURING SEVERITY

*How can you tell how severe your stutter is? What can you use for a baseline measurement?*

We need a standardized scale to measure the degree of severity of your stutter. Dr. Glyndon D. Riley developed such a scale for clinical and research use called the Stuttering Severity Instrument (SSI). Riley described the SSI in the August 1972 issue of the *Journal of Speech and Hearing Disorders* (JSHD). JSHD is a professional journal, so Riley's article was not intended for the average reader. Much of the information in this Step has been rewritten from Riley's article.

## Test Preparation

The SSI yields a single numerical representation of stuttering severity from 0 to 45. Use a sample size of approximately 150 words. The test administration uses two samples, one oral reading sample and one spontaneous speaking sample. For the reading sample, choose a passage of average difficulty for you. You can choose to read from the newspaper, a magazine, or a favorite book. Count out 150 words ahead of time and mark the ending spot. If you do the reading sample first, you will get a feeling for about how many words that is or how long that it takes you. For the spontaneous speaking sample, you speak in your usual way when you speak to a friend. The number of words cannot be counted out ahead of time because this is spontaneous speaking. Allow more time than your reading sample took because you will pause more often to think of what to say. This paragraph is about the right length for a sample.

The recorder should be set up and started before the speaking or reading begins.

## Test Conditions

Try to administer the baseline and each successive test under conditions which are as much alike as possible. This will make your test score comparisons more accurate. This is called "controlling the variables." You want the only change to be the self-therapy so that all differences in scores will reflect the effect of the therapy. Try to administer the tests at about the same time of day, in the same room, with only you and the listener for the spontaneous speaking. Be rested, fed, relaxed. If you are sick, postpone the test a little while so that you can have a chance to recover. All conditions should be as consistently neutral as you can make them. You can even think neutral thoughts to get you in a blank state of mind. You might stutter more if you are tense, excited, upset, etc. Of course, we live in the real world, but if progress shows up under these less stressful conditions, chances are that eventually your stuttering will improve under increasingly stressful conditions.

## Test Administration

Having a helper administer the test is extremely desirable for both accuracy and objectivity. A helper should be relatively easy to obtain, and the majority of you will have tape recorders available to you. Therefore, the test administration will mostly be described assuming these resources. If you are administering the test with different resources, you can adapt the administration to your individual situation. Ideally, the helper could be behind a one-way mirror window with intercom into the test room.

It helps if the tape recorder has a numerical dial. If so, you can number the lines on your recording paper ahead of time. Then record the physical distractions next to the number which corresponds to the number of the tape location as the tape is recording the speech. Then when you listen to the tape and count out the 150 words, you can note the tape location where the sample ends. Find the line on your recording paper with this same numbered tape location and count only distractions recorded before this point. Remember to disregard the first 25 words and then count the next 100 (this leaves out the last 25 also).

If the tape recorder does not have a numerical dial, a stopwatch (or, less easily, a regular watch) could be used. Then you would number the lines on your recording sheet in seconds. After the test, listen to the tape and time the 150-word sample in seconds. Find the line on your recording sheet which corresponds to the time for the sample.

The tape recording will need to be played back several times. You might find it easier to listen for only one aspect at a time.

Observe involuntary actions only, recording:

I. **frequency** of:

    A.  series of *repetitions* of
         sound, syllable, or one-syllable word

Frequency applies to the number of series of repetitions of different sounds. The duration of a series—i.e., the number of repetitions of the same sound in that series—was not recorded, e.g., "M-m-my d-d-dog."

        frequency—2 series of repetitions
(duration would have been—2 series of 3 repetitions each)

Not voluntary repetitions (generally repeated phrases or multiple-syllable words). Rephrasings are also not recorded.

    B.  *prolongation* or position (block)
        1.  silent (non-articulatory)—
          *blocked* pause, not an unblocked pause or
        2.  audible (articulatory)—prolonged sound

II. Record the **duration** of

    *prolongation* of position (block)
        1.  silent (non-articulatory)—
          *blocked* pause, not an unblocked pause or
        2.  audible (articulatory)—prolonged sound

Riley used the average of the *estimates* of the three *longest* blocks as a measure of duration of prolongation. He *estimated* the duration of these blocks so that stopwatch accuracy would not be necessary to maintain reliability. He used the average of the *longest* blocks for greater clinical significance. Longer blocks impede the flow of speech more drastically and so are more easily observed. Reductions in the average duration of these longer blocks makes a more dramatic difference to the stutterer and listener than do reductions of only the shorter average duration of all blocks.

III. Record **frequency, category,** and **location** of

    *concomitants* (distractions)
    A.  audible
    B.  non-audible (silent) physical
        1.  face
        2.  head
        3.  extremities

Here is a somewhat more extensive description of distractions.

A. *Audible.* This category includes any sound which accompanies the stuttered speech. Speech is communication, so it includes language sounds (phonemes) as well as other *voluntary* noises of recognized meaning, such as:

a grunt of disgruntlement or frustration
a snort of indignation

a gasp in shock
a chuckle of delight

a howl of outrage
a squeal of fright
yelp

a groan of despair
a moan of pain

"hmmmm?" in question
"Hmmmmm!" in surprise, satisfaction, or indignation

"unh-hunh" in affirmation
"unhn-uhn" in negation

"a-a-a-h" in relaxation
"Aw-w-w" sheepish embarrassment, disappointment, or pleasure

These sounds are **not** recorded.

Therefore, the only *distractions* are the *involuntary* noises, which have no recognized meaning. These sounds would include:

continual or continued throat clearing
noisy breathing
whistling noises
sniffing (not from cold or sinuses)
blowing
clicking

These sounds count and should be recorded as distractions, even though they are not part of the block itself.

For the severity scores, you must determine the *extent* to which these sounds are distracting to a listener. These judgments are then converted to scores using the scales on the test forms. These scores are what are recorded on the test forms. The location, category, and aspect score subtotals are then added to get the total score.

B. inaudible (silent) physical

1. facial. Usually these distractions are described as grimaces. Any abnormal movement or tension about the face counts in this category. Examples of abnormal facial behavior are:

pressing lips tightly together
tensing jaw muscles
blinking eyes
fluttering eyelids
partially closing eyes
protruding tongue
incoordinated jaw movement

2. head. Generally:

turning head away from the listener to avoid eye contact
looking down at feet
scanning the room
looking up at the ceiling

3. extremities. Any compulsive movement, including

| general body, e.g., | shifting position in the chair |
|---|---|
| specific, e.g., | foot tapping |
| excessive, e.g., | waving hands about the face |
| | wringing the hands |
| | fidgeting with something in the hand |
| | swinging an arm or leg |

*While* you are speaking, i.e., during the observation, not after it, the helper should record a slash mark for each observed disfluency or distraction. In addition, the helper should do the following things in regard to:

1. *prolongations*
   a. estimate duration
   b. convert the estimate to a score between 0 and 9, reflecting the degree of impact the disfluency had on the helper.
   c. record the score directly on the test-form by circling the appropriate number.

*After* the test,

1. Count the frequencies of repetitions, prolongations, and distractions. To count frequencies, skip the first 25 words in the sample. Count the number of stuttered words recorded in the next 100 words of the sample. Bracket the 100 words used. This count is the number of blocks in 100 (a percentage). The table on the test form can be used to convert this percentage into a score. If fewer than 100 words have been spoken, the percentage must be computed. The result of the count converted to a score will yield a numerical value between zero and 9 for each sample, to reach a maximum possible score of 18 for the first aspect.

Record this number in the box to the right of the page marked "Total Frequency Score." The score for "Duration," which has been circled, should be recorded in the box marked "Total Duration Score." The score for distractions is recorded also. The total score is obtained by adding the three subtotals for the aspects.

The SSI can be used when you need to record changes in stuttering severity during the progress of therapy. The single score may suffice to describe overall changes, or each aspect can be treated separately. For example, baseline data for each aspect may be desired when you enter the self-treatment program:

**ASPECTS OF STUTTERING**
**AS MEASURED BY THE**
**STUTTERING SEVERITY INSTRUMENT**
**(SSI)**

| Aspect | Maximum Scores |
|---|---|
| frequency | 18 |
| duration | 7 |
| distractions | 20 |
| Total possible | 45 |

| Degree of Severity | Total Score |
|---|---|
| Very mild | 0–16 |
| Mild | 17–21 |
| Moderate | 22–30 |
| Severe | 31–36 |
| Very severe | 37–45 |

## STUTTERING SEVERITY INSTRUMENT
*Glyndon D. Riley*

**Distractions**

Evaluating Scale:

| Degree of Severity | Score |
|---|---|
| none | 0 |
| not noticeable unless looking for it | 1 |
| barely noticeable to casual observer | 2 |
| distracting | 3 |
| very distracting | 4 |
| severe and painful looking | 5 |

## STUTTERING SEVERITY INSTRUMENT
*Glyndon D. Riley*

**Duration**

| Average of Estimated Length of Three Longest Blocks (Seconds) | Score | |
|---|---|---|
| Fleeting | 1 | |
| 1/2 | 2 | |
| 1 | 3 | Total Duration Score |
| 2–9 | 4 | |
| 10–30 | 5 | |
| 30–60 | 6 | _____ |
| More than 60 | 7 | _____ |

## STUTTERING SEVERITY INSTRUMENT
*Glyndon D. Riley*

**Frequency**

| *Extemporaneous Speaking* | | *Oral Reading* | | |
|---|---|---|---|---|
| *Percentage* | *Score* | *Percentage* | *Score* | |
| 1 | 2 | 1 | 2 | |
| 2–3 | 3 | 2–3 | 2 | |
| 4 | 4 | 4–5 | 5 | |
| 5–6 | 5 | 6–9 | 6 | |
| 7–9 | 6 | 10–16 | 7 | Total Frequency Score |
| 10–14 | 7 | 17–26 | 8 | |
| 15–28 | 8 | 27 and up | 9 | |
| 29 and up | 9 | | | |
| ——— | + | ——— | = | ——— |

*Audible*

| | | | | | | |
|---|---|---|---|---|---|---|
| Noisy breathing whistling sniffing blowing clicking | | 1 | 2 | 3 | 4 | 5 |

*Physical*

| | | | | | | |
|---|---|---|---|---|---|---|
| Facial | — | jaw jerking tongue out lip pressing jaw tense | 1 | 2 | 3 | 4 | 5 |
| Head | — | back forward turning away poor eye contact constant looking around | 1 | 2 | 3 | 4 | 5 |

Total
Distraction
Score

| Extremities — | | 1 | 2 | 3 | 4 | 5 | |
|---|---|---|---|---|---|---|---|
| | arm | | | | | | |
| | hand | | | | | | |
| | fingers | | | | | | _____ |
| | leg | | | | | | |
| | foot | | | | | | |
| | torso | | | | | | _____ |
| | | | | | | | _____ |
| | | | | | | | _____ |

TOTAL SCORE FOR
STUTTERY SEVERITY                    _____

Name _____

Age _____    Gender   M   F

Examined by _____    Date ___/___/___

Progress on each of these parameters could be charted monthly, weekly, or even daily to suit the needs of your program.

    2.  Rank all the prolongations in order of duration. Add the durations of the 3 longest prolongations and average them.

You will find that it is humanly impossible to simultaneously create and observe/score your speech accurately. For the physical distractions, you can try to observe yourself in a mirror, preferably as you are talking to someone in person, less desirably over the telephone, and even less desirably to yourself. Minimally, you need either:

    1.  a tape so that you can create the speech and then observe/listen/ score it/

Tapes of at least the auditory are highly desirable because they can be played back several times to check the accuracy of scoring. They also create a permanent record of your speech at specific dates and stages of therapy. Of course, the physical distractions must be observed visually. Therefore, video recording, if available, is ideal to record all aspects.

    2.  a helper to observe/score the speech while you are creating it.

The initial score and each repeat must be obtained as objectively as possible. In order to obtain reasonably objective scores on the three aspects of stuttering, you may need someone other than yourself to administer the SSI.

If you have access to video recording equipment, a helper can score your speech from a video tape. The next most accurate and objective scoring—and the most likely resources available to you—would be a helper observing/scoring your physical distractions visually in person while an audio tape is made of your speech. The helper then plays back the audio tape several times to score your audible speech and stuttering sounds.

Keep in mind that all conditions of each test administration should be as much alike as possible. This is called "controlling the variables" in an experiment, and it makes the successive scores more comparable. This means that however you decide to do the baseline-original-first-pretherapy administration is how you should do the later administrations, too. This means that if you tape the first administration, the later administrations should be taped.

You may speak differently if you are being taped, or videotaped, or speaking to someone, or over the telephone, or looking in a mirror. Try to make it at the same time of day in the same room with no one else (except the helper) in the room, having eaten and being well rested, feeling well. Keep your speech samples the same length, and of the same approximate difficulty for you. Don't read the same article or repeat a memorized speech, but you could talk about the same subject.

Make a dot for each word spoken fluently and a slash mark for each word stuttered or distraction observed, e.g.,

XXXXXXXXXXXXX

/ . . . / . . / . . . . / . . / . . . . . . /

Remember that any silent or audible prolongation and any repetition of a sound or syllable is considered a stuttered block; whole word and phrase repetitions and rephrasing are not considered blocks.

The monologue should be about a familiar subject such as your job or hobbies. The score for reading aloud can be based on a newspaper item of at least 150 words.

One SSI should be administered before self-therapy begins. After the administration, you should go over your total and aspect scores to see whether you agree that they are true measurements of your stuttering. The scores on that initial administration are your pretherapy or premodification baseline scores. After therapy begins, readminister the SSI at regular intervals, say every three months. The difference between your initial baseline SSI scores and your posttherapy scores measures progress. Comparing your baseline and posttherapy scores in each aspect tells you in what aspect you are improving. Keep in mind that, in the beginning, some scores may actually rise temporarily. Even your total score may rise briefly. Your overall goal is to lower your *total* score with therapy. That is, even if the score for one or two aspects rises, as long as the total score is lowered, you are making progress.

## Step 4

# AN "EASY" APPROACH TO SPEAKING

*What techniques will help you develop an easy approach to stuttering?*

### Relaxation

We all have more difficulty in speaking when we are tense, nervous, or emotional. So, an obvious step in the direction of fluency is relaxation. One author who has written extensively on this subject is Edmund Jacobson, M.D. He developed a method of progressive relaxation which has helped thousands of people to reduce their level of tension. In his book, *You Must Relax* (p. 85), he stated:

> It is physically impossible to be nervous in any part of your body if in that part you are completely relaxed.

Later he gives complete instructions on how to obtain sufficient relaxation.

In talking with stutterers, I have found that a common complaint is "I feel nervous." General relaxation is valuable, but relaxation of the speech muscles is essential. Tension around the face, throat, and chest are very likely to increase your level of stuttering severity. Soft music can be helpful in obtaining a relaxed atmosphere. Closing your eyes and visualizing a quiet lake or other outdoor setting may be your best way of inducing relaxation.

In another book, *Progressive Relaxation,* Jacobson describes in greater detail specific training procedures to induce relaxation. He had his subjects define the tension by first contracting specific muscle groups, beginning, for example, with the toes and working gradually to the head area, and then relaxing them. In the case of stutterers, the most important muscle groups are those involved in speech production.

An early-on advocate of relaxation as an important aspect of therapy for stuttering was Mabel Farrington Gifford. Her method of auto-suggestion, which she learned from Coúe in France, helped her overcome her own severe dysfluency and became the basis for a long career in speech pathology. She believed so sincerely in what she was doing that it almost took on religious dimensions. She was highly successful with stuttering therapy in California and became the first speech pathology consultant in the State Department of Special Education (Murray, 1980, p. 63).

Jacobson writes about two kinds of instructions for procedures in relaxation: "How to relax lying down," and "How to relax while active." In the first procedure, the best position for you is flat on your back; that is, you face the ceiling. Each arm rests directly on the couch in such a way that the hand is at least several inches from the leg. Each portion of the body is supported directly by the couch. Under the conditions stated, you should first get yourself as well relaxed as you can by lying quietly with your eyes open for about three or four minutes, then closing them tightly.

The relaxation procedure progresses as you tense and relax each muscle group. In the procedure for "How to relax while active," the same procedure as that followed while lying down is initiated in a sitting posture, then during activity.

According to Oliver Bloodstein, the relaxation method has a certain basic appropriateness in therapy. He writes that, "It is almost impossible to be relaxed and to stutter in the usual sense at the same time." However, Bloodstein adds, as a result of long experience, considerable dissatisfaction with the relaxation approach has arisen among clinicians. This is based on the evidence that an occasional stutterer seems to learn the trick of relaxing his muscles so effectively that he has little further difficulty with his speech, but such persons appear to be rare. In the usual case, the stutterer tends to speak better in the clinic while practicing relaxation in therapy, but outside the clinic it is not carried over. It is precisely in those situations in which it is most important to do so, anxiety and tension being difficult to separate.

In the book edited by Eisenson, the authors write that they experimented with several types of relaxation, notably those described by Dr. Edmund Jacobson, Mabel Gifford, and a Hindu Yoga variety which consisted of prolonging the exhalation slightly, rolling the eyeballs upward, and contemplating life as a whole. They reported that they were able to produce temporary fluency by these methods, especially when strong suggestion that speech could be fluent was also employed, but this fluency broke down under stress. The authors write, in conclusion, that "to ask a stutterer to relax when he experiences fears of words or audience penalty is to deny the validity of fright" (Eisenson, 1958). Relaxation for a few minutes at the beginning of each therapy session is recommended, but it is not the total answer to an easy approach to speech.

There are cassettes available to encourage relaxation (See Appendix G).

## Rate Control

Parents of young stutterers often insist that the only problem is that the children try to speak too fast. They have observed that if they can get their stuttering children to speak more slowly, they will stutter less or not at all. In general, these parents are correct that an excessive rate is associated with stuttering behavior. Several experts in the area of stuttering have emphasized that slowing down (controlling) the rate of speaking will enhance fluency. Some years ago tremendous claims were made concerning the use of Delayed Auditory Feedback (DAF). This method of therapy utilized an electronic device to control the length of delay between the time the individual spoke into the microphone and received it back into his auditory system. In order to stay with the machine, the speaker had to slow down his speech, for example, to 30 words per minute. Researchers discovered that even severe stutterers could speak fluently if they set the dial to force them to speak slowly enough. In a complete program with DAF, the speaker stays at one level of rate until he is speaking fluently and then changes the dial by 50 millisecond increments until a normal rate is manageable. In most cases, other factors in addition to excessive rate are active so that DAF by itself is inadequate for sustained fluency.

There is no doubt that many stutterers attempt to speak more rapidly than their articulatory skill will tolerate. So, it is highly recommended, especially in the beginning of a therapy program, that rate control be practiced. By experimenting with various rates of speaking, you can determine how slowly you must speak in order to eliminate stuttering. Even though DAF equipment is helpful in establishing the increments in rate, a program of rate control can be initiated and utilized without such equipment.

## Air-Flow Techniques

Many stutterers exhibit *struggle behavior* by trying to force speech out through a contracted, tense speech tract. In the process your vocal chords may be so tense that you prolong sounds, such as "M," "S," or "F," especially at the beginning of words. Your chest muscles might ache with exaggerated efforts to squeeze out speech. Higher up in the speech tract, your articulators—tongue or lips—get "stuck" in position and refuse to progress to the next sound. In this last instance, you either have a silent prolongation (blocking) or you repeat the last sound several times.

Now is the time to practice relaxation and to slow down the rate as much as necessary. A third technique also may be required: air-flow. This technique has been described in detail by Martin Schwartz in his book, *Stuttering Solved.* Many other speech pathologists have advocated its use.

John Addicott, a professor at California State University, Sacramento, California, has written the following:

Among the people talking about air-flow or breathe-out techniques, perhaps the most well-known is Martin Schwartz. In his popular book, *Stuttering Solved,* he gives the world a tantalizing look at the air-flow techniques. These techniques are of interest to me, a speech clinician, primarily because they seem to make the speaking event easier and smoother, with less build up of muscular tension in the muscles of speech. Secondly, these techniques are of interest because many of my stuttering clients appear to have severe blocks occurring at the level of the vocal folds where air-flow techniques can be used most effectively. Some of my stuttering clients seem to use abrupt onsets of voicing and abrupt cessations of voicing even during relative fluent periods of speech. And thirdly, these techniques are of interest because they seem similar to the yawn-sigh techniques which are used during voice therapy to promote usage of the most efficient pitch and to promote smoother, less abrupt, onsets of voicing.

Without providing Dr. Schwartz's controversial explanation for the effectiveness of the air-flow techniques, it is enough to say that many stutterers put their vocal folds under considerable muscular tension. Normally, phonation is achieved by the gentle but rapid vibration of the vocal folds driven by the airstream rising from the lungs. Stutters sometimes tightly squeeze the vocal folds together while pushing the airstream from the lungs vigorously against the vocal folds. They push the air upward by forcibly contracting the muscles of exhalation, primarily the abdominal muscles. In this way, many stutterers make it extremely difficult to get phonation started and to keep the phonation going. Excessive tension and effort is not an efficient nor an effective way to do voicing and to do speaking. Instead of pushing harder to blast through a perceived blockage at the vocal folds, it would be more effective for the stutterer to reduce the muscular tension of the vocal folds and to allow the vocal folds to be vibrated easily by the upward movement of the airstream. It would also be more effective for the stutterer to create the upward movement of the airstream by gradually relaxing the muscles of inhalation instead of by forcefully contracting the muscles of exhalation. The term "passive" flow is sometimes used to talk about the upward movement of the airstream being provided by the gradual relaxation of the muscles of inhalation.

The air-flow techniques seem to be excellent ways to teach stutterers how to reduce the muscular tension and how to prevent the muscular tension from building up. Basically, in these techniques, the stuttering client is instructed to take a normal inhalation, then start an easy exhalation by gradually relaxing the muscles of inhalation. This easy exhalation prevents the vocal folds from closing tightly and prevents the vocal folds from becoming highly tense. The easy exhalation prevents the abdominal muscles from becoming as very tense as they can when they are pushing against closed vocal folds. Then, without stopping the easy exhalation or only minimally interrupting the easy exhalation, the stutterer begins to speak.

In addition to requiring flow of breath before speaking, the air-flow techniques also require an on-going easiness about speaking. Muscular tension cannot be allowed to build up at any time during speech. The phrase "passive flow, soft and slow" can be used as a reminder (Schwartz, 1976, p. 116).

Initially, the air-flow techniques can be practiced in single words. Be sure you observe a clear indication of an easy passive air-flow or exhalation. Then the techniques build toward longer and longer phrases on a passive exhalation. Practice continues in the more difficult and more complex speaking situations the stutterer will be encountering.

For some stutterers, the easy exhalation or the slight flow of air before speaking may become shorter and shorter. Sometimes the air-flow may seem to fade out completely, making this technique resemble what Van Riper described as a prepatory set not to stutter. However, I think it would be wiser for a stuttering client to maintain the brief passive exhalation of air before beginning the speaking attempt so that this air-flow tool will be familiar and frequently used. Then when the client is in a very difficult speaking situation, the tool will be readily available to him or her.

There are a number of benefits to using an air-flow technique. One of these is that fluent speech can be achieved in some situations relatively easily and quickly. The stuttering clients are encouraged that changes are possible and that success is possible. They are encouraged to attempt other changes and accomplish even greater successes. Many of the clients find the normalness of the resulting speech is desirable and they are willing to work toward the new speaking style. The mental imagery that is used to teach air-flow techniques may be very helpful for the clients to remember in the difficult speaking situations the clients may find themselves. The easy exhalation before starting a word gives information to the client and to the clinician that the client is actually ready to start the word in an easy, smooth manner.

I have also observed a number of very serious problems with the air-flow techniques. One of these may occur when clients are not fully aware or fully instructed on using the techniques. The clients may push the exhalation too hard and find it is not effective. They may find that they are still stuttering. Their incorrect use of the air-flow technique very quickly may become part of their secondary package of stuttering behaviors.

A second problem is that the apparent success and the good feelings that are being generated by being fluent may promote a high degree of fluency. Being successful may promote fluency and the clients may not learn the techniques very well. The clients may not realize they do not know the techniques very well for quite a period of time. They may not realize it until they are out of therapy.

A third problem that greatly concerns me is that by promoting fluent speech, the clinician may be supporting and reinforcing the clients' long standing desires to be fluent speakers and may be supporting their unrealistic expectations to have perfectly fluent speech. I think it is important for stutterers to realize that not all disfluencies are equal. There are some that occur for thinking and swallowing. Some occur for breathing and some for emphasis. Some occur for planning word choice and for planning articulation. These disfluencies need to be tolerated and used by the clients to prepare their ideas and their speech mechanisms. Some more severe disfluencies may precipitate a painful reaction or a panic reaction. Perhaps these latter disfluencies can only be accepted or tolerated as mere happenings. Perhaps a client needs to realize that a successful life continues beyond the disfluency. That is very easy for me to say, but it may be very necessary for some clients to learn.

In summary, I have tried to show some of the basic ideas behind some of the air-flow techniques. What I have related is not enough to be used without considerable study and practice. In addition, I have tried to show some of the benefits of the air-flow techniques and I have tried to show some of the very serious problems.

# Step 5

# ELIMINATING "TRICKS"

*What behaviors have I been using to cover-up or postpone stuttering?*

You must make a real effort to identify and eliminate, that means stop, all avoidance, substitution, or postponement habits which you have accumulated over the years to put off or hide your stuttering. Although these behaviors supply temporary relief, they actually increase your fears and cause you more trouble in the long run.

The more you make a practice of avoiding, postponing, or substituting, and the more you keep on using such crutches, you reinforce your fear of stuttering. Avoidance tactics include dodging speaking situations, avoiding social contacts, or talking on the telephone. Postponements may be repeating words, going back to get a running start or clearing the throat unnecessarily. Playing dumb or hard-of-hearing are also examples of postponement devices. Additionally, you might use interjections like, "uh," "well," or "now, let's see." Substitutions involve using synonyms, easy words, or other word phrases for those on which you think you might block. So, if you willingly adopt an attitude of *not* trying to cover-up or avoid, you have made a giant step toward fluency (Fraser, #12, p. 8).

As soon as you become aware of any of the above mentioned behaviors, concentrate on eliminating them one by one. Don't postpone getting started; do it now. For example, instead of acting as though you didn't hear or understand a question, answer in the best manner you can. As a teacher, I have observed many stutterers who mumble "I don't know" when they do know. They may give a truncated answer, but it is better for everyone concerned than an untruthful failure to respond.

You can record in a notebook examples of your avoidance, postponements, and substitutions with tally marks to make you fully aware of how often they occur. At first, you may prefer to make your notation in secret; later, you may do it openly. Then, if anyone asks what you are doing, you can answer, "I'm working on my speech problem."

Charles Van Riper (1982, pp. 131–133) describes avoidance and postponement behaviors in detail. *Refusal behavior* is utilized when the stutterer refuses to enter communication situations in which he expects to stutter, or he refuses to attempt certain feared words. Many stutterers feign stupidity in school to avoid reciting and others pretend to be deaf so they can write out what they have to say. Most frequent of all refusal behaviors are those involving substitutions and circumlocutions. A side effect is that some stutterers develop a large vocabulary in their search for synonyms or alternate ways to get across their messages. Stutterers may adopt a sing-song type of speech or chant their words. Some speak very rapidly and run their words together as though they are afraid to pause.

Delaying the attempt to speak is accomplished by using postponement techniques. Normal speakers use "ahs," "ers," or repeat phrases as they decide how to say what they have to say. Stutterers use these same strategies and many others. Some stutterers postpone silently and then blurt out the word or phrase. With continued use, these behaviors become automatic and interfere with oral communication without the knowledge of the stutterers. If at all possible, you may need the assistance of a sympathetic friend in locating avoidances and postponement behaviors. Sooner or later, unless they disappear spontaneously, they must be identified and eliminated.

Step 6

# ELIMINATING SECONDARY
# PHYSICAL CHARACTERISTICS

*How can you become aware of secondary physical behaviors? Can you set up
a program to eliminate them?*

This step in the process toward fluency is similar to Step 5 except that
the "enemy" is more noticeable to the listener. These "with-movements"
may have become so habituated that you are not aware that they occur
but most of them can rarely be hidden. Of course, some of them, such as
crunching of the toes or making a fist in your coat pocket can be
unobserved, but facial contortions, flailing of the arms, or stamping of
the feet become obvious. It is possible that you have no such irregular
behaviors, but most stutterers do.

These movements include eye blinks, nostril or facial grimaces, mouth
protrusions or postures, and the like. In the summer of 1988, the movie,
*A Fish Called Wanda*, caused controversy in part because of the portrayal
of a severe stutterer in one of the leading roles. This character had
numerous secondary physical movements which were unnecessary for
the production of speech. Typical of many stutterers, the number and
intensity of these behaviors increased with the degree of emotional
involvement. The actor did an excellent job of giving a realistic picture
of a severe stutterer under such environmental pressures. Some critics
gave the movie high ratings while others thought it was cruel to animals,
women, and stutterers. The goals for this book do not include such
discussions, but we all must be aware of the listener's reactions to the
various problems of the stutterer.

In your program to overcome these extraneous movements, you can
ask a trusted friend to watch when you are speaking and report his
observations to you. You need to raise to the level of consciousness any
unnecessary movements you make when stuttering or anticipating
stuttering. Speaking before a full length mirror will be beneficial in the
process of identification. An example would be observing yourself in a
mirror as you talk on the telephone.

One of the most important aspects of successful oral communication is maintaining adequate eye contact with the listener. Rather than looking at the floor, ceiling, or into the distance, you must establish direct eye contact and maintain it for reasonable periods of time. This doesn't mean that you need to stare fixedly at the person, but you should maintain eye contact more or less continuously. Particularly do your best not to look away when you stutter or expect to. You might ask someone with whom you converse to report on whether you shift your eyes just before or when you stutter (Fraser, 1980, p. 95).

Start by looking at yourself in a mirror and faking an easy block. Try this repeatedly, making sure that you don't look away. Make some phone calls while looking at yourself even while you are having real blocks. While talking to others note your successes in maintaining eye contact. Write down the names of individuals with whom you were successful and/or write down ten or more words on which you stuttered without losing eye contact. Build confidence in your ability to speak with good natural eye contact on all occasions. It will give you satisfaction to know that you can maintain eye contact and it will make you a more effective conversationalist.

Step 7

# NEGATIVE EMOTIONS

*What are negative emotions? How can you control them?*

There is difference of opinion among speech therapists about when, in a program to overcome dysfluency, is the best time to attack this problem of negative emotions. From my experience, I have concluded that negative emotions, such as anger, guilt, shame, embarrassment, and frustration, often diminish in intensity or disappear entirely as fluency improves. In those cases in which such spontaneous improvement is not forthcoming, a more direct approach is necessary.

As early as 1957, C.S. Bluemel included information about the personality and emotional tolerance of stutterers in his book, *The Riddle of Stuttering.* Contrary to some other researchers, he maintained that personality traits were the cause rather than the result of stuttering.

> As a person, the stutterer is often diffident, sensitive, self-conscious, indecisive, tense, and easily confused. It is difficult to find one who is well organized, or one who is bold and extroverted. The average stutterer has difficulty with his social adjustments, and when he fails to express himself, it is because his weak ego makes him hesitant and uncertain. Personal relations torment the stutterer. At a dinner party, he may speak fluently while the cocktails are being served, and while people are talking informally and moving about, but he is likely to have trouble when he takes his place at the table and is confronted by strangers (p. 65).

He adds:

> The pattern of frustration and disorganization is not confined to speech; it is seen in many learning processes. He has difficulty in learning to play a piano, operating a typewriter, or driving an automobile. In these situations, over-eagerness, timidity or anxiety tends to defeat the learning process. Embarrassment in social situations leads to disorganizations in many patterns. Functional skills are not easily learned by tense and timid people, and this applies to speech. In the broad medical concept, the riddle of stuttering involves a good deal more than speech. It involves the stutterer's personality, his native non-fluency, his environmental stress, his disorganization in the sphere of speech, his struggle with the speech block, and his conditioning

experiences. Manifestly, the treatment of stuttering requires more than "speech correction." It calls for a broad psychological approach (p. 69).

One way to begin overcoming emotional upsets is to create a hierarchy of speaking situations and then attack them in order of difficulty from easy to difficult. A high school stutterer composed the following list.

1. Speaking out loud to myself when alone.
2. Speaking to pets or animals.
3. Speaking to babies or young children.
4. Speaking to older children.
5. Speaking to my mother.
6. Speaking to fellows my age.
7. Speaking to girls my age.
8. Speaking to my father.
9. Speaking to women I don't know.
10. Speaking to men I don't know.
11. Speaking to store clerks.
12. Speaking before a group who knows me.
13. Speaking before a group who doesn't know me.
14. Speaking on the telephone to a friend.
15. Speaking on the telephone to a stranger.

(Speech Foundation of America, #10, 1974, p. 68)

Frederick Murray relates that the playwright Thornton Wilder gave him three bits of advice.

1. Stop worrying about yourself and your stuttering. You are focusing too much on that.
2. Find some kind of endeavor that you can throw yourself into, that is beyond you, that is creative, and in which you are doing something to help other people.
3. Hang onto your sense of humor.

Fred considered the advice about humor to be the most significant (1980, p. 53).

You can get some notion of your personality patterns by putting a check mark on each of the following lines which connect pairs of opposing adjectives.

1. Shy. . . . . . . . . . . . . . . . . . . . . . . . . . . . . . . . . . . bold
2. Anxious . . . . . . . . . . . . . . . . . . . . . . . . . . . . . composed
3. Unfriendly. . . . . . . . . . . . . . . . . . . . . . . . . . . . friendly
4. Hesitant . . . . . . . . . . . . . . . . . . . . . . . . . . . . . daring
5. Fearful. . . . . . . . . . . . . . . . . . . . . . . . . . . . . . fearless
6. Unpleasant . . . . . . . . . . . . . . . . . . . . . . . . . . . pleasant
7. Nervous. . . . . . . . . . . . . . . . . . . . . . . . . . . . . . calm
8. Tense. . . . . . . . . . . . . . . . . . . . . . . . . . . . . . . relaxed
9. Insecure . . . . . . . . . . . . . . . . . . . . . . . . . . . . . secure
10. Afraid . . . . . . . . . . . . . . . . . . . . . . . . . . . . . . confident

In a study done at the University of Alabama by Eugene Fowlie and Eugene Cooper, mothers of stuttering children described their children as being more anxious, introverted, fearful, sensitive, withdrawn, and insecure than the answers supplied by mothers of nonstuttering children. Whether such results would occur with adults is unknown. There is need for further research.

Another approach to coping with negative emotions is to study your emotional reaction before, during, and after episodes of stuttering. What circumstances trigger moments of stuttering and how do you react to them? When, for example, does tension mount and burst forth with feelings of anxiety: before, during, or after a moment of stuttering? The same observation needs to made in regard to anger, guilt, and frustration. Who, you or your listener, is responsible for negative reactions? How often do these negative feelings occur? Once an hour, twice a week, three times a month, etc.?

How have you been coping with these negative emotions? Refusal to try again, crying, maintaining a brooding silence, or what else? In most instances, your listener is understanding and waits for you to make the next move. Or, can you learn to say, "I'm having a little trouble. I'll try again."

Perhaps the *Credo* developed by Jack Carlisle would be helpful (p. 144).

## The Stutterer's Credo

I believe that I can maintain fluent speech provided that I *prolong* my words and *speak slowly* at a rate I can manage.
I use *voluntary controlled repetition* to signal people that I stutter and to help me past potential blocks;
I approach the beginning of words *gently* and slowly,
I *never push past blocks;*
I *pause (i.e., cancel) when I block,* and try again, approaching the word

slowly and smoothly, using voluntary controlled repetition when necessary;

I *never* try to avoid a block by *substituting* an easy word for a hard word;

I *remain in contact* with the audience and myself, and keep sufficient eye contact not to cause embarrassment;

I *never hide my stutter* from myself or other people;

I *practice* good speech technique as often as possible in order to stutter in a fluent manner that will not interrupt communication.

I added another component later: "I shall *never* lose my temper with people who react rudely to my stuttering and, for the sake of other stutterers, I must *never* let them get away with it."

Emotional habits, like other human reactions, do not change rapidly. If your ability to cope with the negative emotion associated with stuttering has not improved within a year, it would be advisable to seek professional help in the area of psychotherapy. Research shows that such professional assistance probably will not change your problem of dysfluency, but it may improve your chances for success in a program aimed specifically at improving fluency. Although both programs can be undertaken concurrently, it is often advisable to discontinue the speech program until the program in psychotherapy is completed.

Step 8

# SPECIAL TECHNIQUES FOR ENHANCING FLUENCY

Charles Van Riper has explained in depth the use of cancellations, pull-outs, and prepatory sets in a number of publications, including his text book, *Treatment of Stuttering*. A simplified explanation of these special techniques has been published by the Speech Foundation of America in the fourth edition of Publication #12, *Self-therapy for the Stutterer*.

**Cancellations**

When you stutter on a word, put into action the following sequence.

1. Finish the word on which you had difficulty.
2. Pause—come to a complete stop, once the word has been uttered. The pause is to give you time to study your problem and pantomime its solution.
3. Try to relax the tension in your speech mechanism, throat, tongue and lips. The key is to feel the tension draining out as your breathing returns to normal.
4. Think back and ask yourself what caused you to get stuck.
5. Review what you can do to slowly reverse or change the errors you made on this particular sound or word.
6. Mentally rehearse or silently mimic how it feels to have your mouth slowly make these corrections so as to modify your usual pattern of stuttering and move through the word.
7. Repeat the word as you feel yourself making the corrections.
8. Articulate the sound on which you blocked in a slow motion, prolonged manner.

Although this postblock correction may seem to take a long time, it will take only a few seconds. The slow, prolonged way of working your way through the word will give you plenty of time to feel yourself making the corrections.

**Pull-Outs**

After you have learned to use cancellations, you can use a somewhat comparable method of pulling out of a block when you are in the midst of one. Rather than struggling blindly, trying to force your way out, it would be better to use a systematic method.

When you find yourself in the middle of a block, don't pause and don't stop and try again. Instead, continue the stuttering, slowing it down and letting the block run its course. Deliberately make a smooth prolongation of what you are doing. You will be stabilizing the sound by slowing down a repetition, or changing the repetition to a prolongation, or smoothing out a tremor or pulling out of a fixation as you ease out of the block.

Hold the stuttering long enough to feel control and figure out what you are doing wrong and what needs to be done to change your faulty actions. Then voluntarily release yourself by discontinuing the prolongation or repetitions. If you fail to move out of the block, do a postblock cancellation in order to keep the feeling of being in control.

**Preparatory Set**

Before using this technique, you should be adept at correcting your stuttering after it happens. You now need to learn how to make preparations to forestall your stuttering before it happens. You need to learn *pre*block correction.

You can take advantage of the fact that you usually anticipate difficulty before it happens. You can learn how to cope with your stuttering by "moving out" ahead of a block and approaching it with preblocking corrections. They are similar to postblock corrections except that your planning is done *before* rather than *after* the need arises.

Here is the sequence of actions on your part when you approach a feared sound or word.

1. Pause—come to a complete stop. The pause will not be long, but this willingness to stop will convince both you and your listener that you are determined to be in control of the situation.
2. Try to relax the tensed area of your speech mechanism, including your throat, tongue, and lips.
3. Recall what you usually do abnormally when you block on that sound or word.

4. Figure out what corrections you have learned to change what you usually did wrong.
5. Rehearse in your mind, or actually pantomime how it would feel in your mouth to put these corrections into effect.
6. Say the word, making the corrections as you rehearsed them. Articulate the sound and word in a sliding, resonant, prolonged manner. Pay more attention to how the word feels than how it sounds.

These techniques can be useful whenever dysfluencies (moments of stuttering) occur. They must be mastered in private and kept in readiness for unexpected relapses. They are the threads in your security blanket.

# Step 9

# CARRY-OVER

*Are you ready to participate in speaking situations in the "real world"? Are you willing to seek out and initiate conversational possibilities? Are you ready to join the National Stuttering Project (NSP)?*

To a greater or lesser degree, you may have been working on your stuttering in the privacy of your "closet." Now it is time to emerge and make an all out effort to apply what you have been practicing. Rather than avoiding speaking situations, you must seek out opportunities to speak. You must, if necessary, adopt an aggressive approach toward starting conversations in one-on-one situations. Rather than merely saying, "Hi," you must gradually add information or questions to lengthen your oral contacts with the people in your environment.

You are now ready to make your own hierarchy of speaking situations which become your immediate and long-term goals for improved fluency. Tackle the easier ones immediately and work up (or down) to the more difficult ones gradually. Don't try to rush progress; be reasonable in your expectations. Frederick Murray relates his sad experience in accepting an invitation to speak at a national conference of the American Speech Language and Hearing Association (ASHA) in Chicago before he was ready for such an assignment. His expectations were very high but unrealistic. He writes as follows:

> When my turn came and I reached the podium, I opened my mouth and went immediately into tremors. I had almost no control. Besides the tremors, I was battling severe blockages that I could not seem to pull out of. The more I tried to prevent their happening, the worse they were. Somehow, I struggled on even though the ghastly tremors and the blocking continued. At last, I blurted out the final word and sat down, burning with shame (p. 129).

He did recover and eventually, with a Ph.D. from the University of Denver in Speech Pathology, he became a professor at the University of New Hampshire. Over the years he gained increased control over his fluency problem and is now recognized as a national authority on stuttering. Success was delayed, however, while he practiced diligently on less pressureful speaking situations. So, start at the bottom of the ladder and climb slowly, but resolutely to the top. As you conquer each level of speaking situations, go on to the next. The fluency checklist in Appendix C can suggest possibilities for your personal hierarchy of speaking situations. Each stutterer has his own fears, so that a speaking situation which is easy for one stutterer is very difficult for another and vice versa. Make your own priority list and get busy.

Planning, practicing, and taking notes might require a minimum of an hour each day. But, if you are serious about improvement in fluency, do it. Musicians, athletes, and others make far greater commitments to obtain their goals.

As you are successful with more complicated speaking situations, you may want to consider joining the local chapter of the National Stuttering Project (NSP). More details are given about this self-help organization for stutterers in Appendix F. If there is no such organization in your community, why not contact the national office in San Francisco and get one started. Stuttering, you know by this time, is your problem, so your next step could be helping to establish a local chapter of NSP.

Such groups have been formed throughout the United States by the National Stuttering Project (NSP). Here, stutterers can apply newly developed fluency skills with sympathetic listeners. Members of the group make suggestions for coping with various speech situations, based on their own experiences in trying to overcome stuttering. For further details about the organization, see Appendix F.

Joseph Sheehan spent many years as a faculty member in psychology at the University of California, Los Angeles developing techniques of group therapy for adult stutterers. He published numerous articles about his theories and methods as well as editing *Stuttering: Research and Theory,* 1970.

Features of Group Therapy (Sheehan, 1970)

1. Stutterers can do things for each other in groups that cannot be accomplished in individual therapy.
2. The group situation is in itself a facsimile of social interaction, the area in which most of the stutterer's interpersonal difficulties reside.
3. Through group tolerance, understanding and support, important forces are available to promote growth in the stutterer.
4. Related to the above is that initiative may be originated or inspired in a group experience. The stutterer may find that he has increased courage to do things among an accepting, supportive group.

5. The group provides a relatively safe place for the stutterer to attempt new ways of behaving.
6. Part of most stuttering therapies consist of discovering stuttering patterns and underlying attitudes. Sharing with others aids in opening up this process.
7. The individual members of the group not only learn from each other new approaches to the solutions of their problems, they also assume the role of therapist for other members and finally for themselves.

Charles Van Riper, after obtaining a Ph.D. in Speech Pathology at the University of Iowa, spent his entire professional life as a faculty member at Western Michigan University. He, too, was convinced of the benefits of group therapy for stutterers. He was aware, in addition, of some of the pitfalls of the group situation.

Difficulties and Disadvantages of Group Therapy (Van Riper, 1973)

1. Often times the composition of the group may be too heterogeneous to facilitate interaction or may contain exploiters and saboteurs.
2. At times unhealthy attitudes may become contagious.
3. Some members who most need to participate may remain on the fringes of the group and stay uninvolved.
4. The group may become a safe harbor and refuge and prevent the person from making the adjustment to reality.
5. Certain members may be overwhelmed by group pressures for disclosure of events and feelings and either leave the group or become shattered.
6. Group therapy requires a very skilled and competent leader, and there aren't many of them.

# Step 10

# TRYING PUBLIC SPEAKING

*Have you always avoided speaking to groups of half a dozen or more individuals? Have you asked friends to substitute for you in such situations? Has such behavior been a disadvantage to your social or professional life?*

In most cases, stutterers have refused to try public speaking situations, such as giving announcements, taking part in panel discussions, or presenting projects before a class. One client I had recently had successfully avoided all such public presentation until his senior year in college when he was required to give an oral report in an engineering class. He blocked severely and was unable to complete the report. So he decided to seek professional help in speech therapy. The techniques which he learned in six therapy sessions made it possible for him to present his report before the class with only minimal difficulty.

When fluency has progressed adequately, stutterers are encouraged to take classes in public speaking either in college or in nationally known commercial courses, such as those offered by Dale Carnegie. Another source of practice are the Toastmaster International Clubs which are available in most cities throughout the United States. Then, of course, local professional and social clubs give opportunities for public speaking activities. Reading the scripture in church is another possibility. Stutterers whose severity is moderate or less might volunteer in fund raising campaigns and political events.

Basic to success in public speaking, as well as in one-on-one situations, is to have something interesting to say. You may need to expand your interests and areas of expertise so that the subjects of your presentations are worthwhile to the audience. A dull person is more likely to fail before a group. Skill in public speaking develops with practice. Stage fright, a common enemy of early attempts at public speaking, tends to disappear with improvement in self-confidence.

One noted example of a person who started out as a poor public speaker and, through continued effort and specific training, became an outstanding success was Eleanor Roosevelt. What she did, many of us, including stutterers, can do.

72

If you live near a community college or university, enrolling in a beginning course in public speaking should be considered. However, you need to feel ready for such an adventure. Unfortunately, not all instructors are kindly in their criticism nor helpful in their suggestions. If possible, you might want to check with students who have taken their classes. This is a vital step for your program in overcoming dysfluencies. You cannot be too cautious.

# Step 11

# EVALUATING YOUR LIFE STYLE

*Do you follow a lifestyle that permits improvements in fluency? Is your life so filled with nonessential activities that a sense of calm is missing? If so, what factors in the environment and in your attitudes need changing?*

It is difficult for stutterers to remain calm and relaxed when their lifestyles are hectic. Some stutterers are high-strung and attempt to compensate for their speech shortcomings by a frantic social and/or professional life. There may be need for compromise. You should examine your schedule of social and work events to determine if you need to cut out some of the superfluous activities. Serenity is hard to come by in an overcrowded, overscheduled regime.

So you must look realistically at your schedule. Are you trying to do too many things? Are you putting too much pressure on yourself to achieve near perfection in too many areas? Work toward a well balanced schedule of work, exercise, and entertainment. And, of course, provide adequate time for rest. Learn to say, "No" to demands for more commitments on your time and energy.

As you develop what is for you a satisfying, nonpressuring routine, you will find that your fluency improves. Don't conclude that "routine" is dull, but that organization of time and energy is a sensible approach for everyone, especially stutterers.

Take time to make a list of your activities for one week. Examine the list to determine what can be eliminated. You may find that a third of the things you do could be tossed away without injury to your professional or social life. In addition, consider replacing some hectic, tension-producing activities with slower-paced, less tenseful activities. How often, for example, do you take a leisurely walk before bedtime?

Another area of exploration is your collection of personality traits. By the time you are an adult, these reactions to events and interpersonal relations have become habituated. Do you like and admire the type of person you have become? If you had a choice, would you choose yourself (a person like you) as a best friend?

Bluemel (p. 64) has described the personality of the stutterer.

As a person, he is often diffident, sensitive, selfconscious, indecisive, tense, and easily confused . . . The stammerer appears to be a low dominance person in a culture where high dominance is prevalent.

In the broad medical concept, the riddle of stammering involves a good deal more than speech. It involves the stammerer's personality, his native nonfluency, his environmental stresses, his disorganization in the sphere of speech, his struggle with the speech block, his conditioning experiences, and the final phase of phobia. Manifestly, the treatment of stammering requires something more than "speech correction." It calls for a broad psychological approach. It is altogether likely that a permanent change in fluency may require a change in you.

One way of beginning a serious study of yourself is to write an autobiography. You may discover that you have been more responsible for what has happened to you than you realized. The tendency is for individuals to feel that they are victims of circumstances beyond their control. No doubt, in some cases, that is true, but is it true in your case?

Your autobiography might emphasize that period of your life beyond age 21. The older you are, the more years have been available for you to take charge of your life. As with stuttering, your basic problems are a reflection of your lifestyle. In recent years, how have you handled the negative emotions of frustration, hostility, and shame?

Albert Murry, in the Foundation of Speech series #10, *Therapy for Stutterers* (p. 99), 1974 has written the following:

What does it take to speak? What enhances speech regardless of social or therapeutic setting? Our observations convince us that the following conditions contribute to the stutterer's speaking ability:

1. Whatever helps the client feel freer, share himself, and affect others in socially desirable ways.
2. Whatever helps the client come closer to others, touch them and be touched in any humanizing sense.
3. Whatever helps the client live with greater joyful spontaneity, nonverbally and verbally.
4. Whatever increases his feelings of hope, faith, and trust, in others and in himself.
5. Whatever increases his willingness to risk complete living, the courage to be himself fully.
6. Whatever increases his feelings of personal worth, and his ability to love and be loved.

# Step 12

## ACCEPTING FLUENCY

*Do you feel that your improvement in fluency is a fluke? Are there times when your lack of stuttering frightens you?*

Stutterers find it necessary to adjust to fluency. You must learn to accept your role as a nearly normal speaker. Secondary gains, such as being excused from your share in money raising campaigns, giving class reports, or taking part in panel discussions are no longer legitimate. Another adjustment is accepting yourself as an ex-stutterer who is capable of speech within normal limits.

In the days when your stuttering was a real problem, you may have blamed your disfluency for many of your social and professional failures. Now, as a more nearly normal speaker, you still have areas of failure in your personal and professional life. In other words, the stuttering itself was *not* the cause of poor interpersonal relationships or lack of promotion at work. It is not easy to accept this conclusion and look for other causes. We all, of course, have personality factors which hold us back in our social or work endeavors. And, now that disfluencies are no longer a significant problem, can you find other reasons that your family life, for example, does not run along as smoothly as you would like? Possibly you have been too perfectionistic and, as a result, have set unrealistic standards of behavior for yourself and other members of your family. Another example, you might have been too sensitive to remarks made by persons in your work situation and taken them personally. Stutterers, as a group, tend to overreact when joking remarks are made in their presence. Learn to say, "What do you mean?" or "Please explain that to me?" rather than take personal offence and carry a grudge. The speaker might have been joking or sounding sarcastic without intending to "cut you down."

Joseph Sheehan (p. 294) has made a summary statement concerning adjusting to fluency.

*Adjusting to Fluency.* You may be astonished that fluency is anything to which you would have to adjust. Yet it is a central problem in the consolidation of improvement. Just as in the early phases of therapy, you had to accept your role as a stutterer, so in the later phases, you have to accept your role as a more normal speaker. The second adjust-ment is sometimes bigger than the first one. You have to overcome the feeling that all fluency is false and undeserved. You may even need to accept the responsibility and disappointment that result when you learn that your conquest of stuttering does not magically solve every other problem in life.

# Step 13

## COPING WITH RELAPSE

*Does a "bad day" discourage you? Are you able to apply special techniques to get yourself going again?*

Although very few research studies about stuttering therapy include data about relapse, we are aware that relapse does occur. It is frustrating to the stutterer when his disfluencies increase and he feels that his level of disfluency is greater than it was three or six months previously. We all know, of course, that success in most of life's endeavors are not constantly uphill, but that "down periods" do occur. In stuttering, such relapse periods may last for a day, week, or month before improvement is again significant.

According to Franklin H. Silverman, who wrote an article about "Relapse Following Stuttering Therapy," the main reason for relapse is that stutterers "forget" to do what was prescribed by their clinicians. They may get so busy in the professional and social aspects of life, that lack of fluency is no longer a priority.

So what is to be done? If relapse should occur, you will need to repeat the steps toward improved fluency as outlined in this book. No doubt you will be able to reach levels of adequate fluency much more quickly the second time. In any event, you will need to back up at least to Step Three and reevaluate your level of disfluency. Take the time and effort to restudy your present stuttering pattern and then go through the various steps as outlined. There is no need to cry. Just try again.

There is a natural tendency to return to old habits, such as using avoidance or denying your stuttering. Sometimes you may have a "bad day" for no apparent reason, so you need to accept these conditions as normal and not dwell upon them. Don't expect perfection as such an attitude builds up pressure and leads to more "struggle behavior."

In the Speech Foundation of America publication, *Self-Therapy for the Stutterer,* Malcolm Fraser suggests the following ground rules. Compare them to the steps that have been recommended in this book.

Rule  1—Talking slowly and deliberately
Rule  2—Stuttering easily
Rule  3—Admitting that you stutter
Rule  4—Eliminating avoidances, postponements and substitutions
Rule  5—Eliminating secondary symptoms
Rule  6—Maintaining eye contact
Rule  7—Finding out what you do when you stutter
Rule  8—Block corrections
Rule  9—Using inflections
Rule 10—Listening to your fluent speech
Rule 11—Talking all you can

If you become discouraged with your progress toward acceptable fluency, consider professional help. Contact the American Speech-Language-Hearing Association, 10801 Rockville Pike, Rockville, Maryland, 20852.

# FINAL EXAMINATION

Now that you have worked your way through the 13 steps toward improvement in fluency, here is the final examination. Can you answer *Yes* to each of the following statements?

Yes—No 1. I am willing to declare openly that I have difficulty with fluency.

Yes—No 2. I assume responsibility for my stuttering problem without blaming other people.

Yes—No 3. I have made overcoming my stuttering a first priority and plan to do so indefinitely.

Yes—No 4. I have learned to listen to myself in order to study my pattern of disfluencies.

Yes—No 5. I can use the *Stuttering Severity Index* by Dr. Glyndon Riley to determine my improvement in fluency.

Yes—No 6. I constantly apply relaxation techniques as a first step in an easy approach to speaking.

Yes—No 7. I can control my rate of speaking and slow down whenever I have difficulties with fluency.

Yes—No 8. I can apply air-flow techniques in times of disfluency.

Yes—No 9. I have been able to eliminate "tricks" to hide my occasional moments of stuttering.

Yes—No 10. I have discontinued the use of "secondaries," such as finger tapping or head jerking.

Yes—No 11. I have made a conscious effort to obtain and maintain eye contact with my listeners.

Yes—No 12. I have learned to control my emotional reactions to stuttering episodes.

Yes—No 13. I have learned to use cancellations, pull-outs, and preparatory sets whenever they are needed.

Yes—No 14. I have been able to transfer these skills in speaking to real-life situations.

Yes—No 15.  I have participated in self-help groups for stutterers.
Yes—No.16.  I have accepted opportunities to speak before groups of people.
Yes—No 17.  I have enrolled in a public speaking class.
Yes—No 18.  I have examined my life-style and made changes which are beneficial to my level of fluency.
Yes—No 19.  I no longer use my stuttering problem as an excuse for nonparticipation in social or professional assignments.
Yes—No 20.  I can recognize periods of relapse as "normal procedure" and apply whatever parts of the program are appropriate to regain a higher level of fluency.

How did you come out? Using 1 for Yes and 0 for No, a possible grading scale could be:

$$18-20 \quad A$$
$$15-17 \quad B$$
$$12-14 \quad C$$
$$9-11 \quad D$$
$$\text{Below } 9 \quad F$$

If you came out with a poor grade, perhaps you didn't make this project high enough on your list of "to do" activities. More time, effort, and concentration might bring better results.

A second possibility is that you need professional guidance in working on your stuttering problem. In this case, the American Speech-Language-Hearing Association has a list of certified speech therapists throughout the United States. The special education division of local city or county schools may be helpful in locating a qualified speech therapist.

In any event, don't give up! All stutterers can be helped to improve their oral communication skills. The vast majority can reach a level of fluency so that stuttering is no longer a significant factor in their personal and professional life.

## REFERENCES

### (Books)

Barbara, Dominick, *New Directions in Stuttering.* Charles C Thomas, Publisher: Springfield, IL, 1965.

Bloodstein, Oliver, *Stuttering in Speech Pathology: An Introduction* (Second Edition). Houghton Mifflin Company: Boston, 1984.

Bluemel, C.S., *The Riddle of Stuttering*. Interstate Publishing Company: Danville, IL, 1957.

Boberg, Einer (Editor), *Maintenance of Fluency*. Elsevier: New York, 1981.

Bryngelson, Bryng, Myfanwy E. Chapmand and Orvetta K. Hansen, *Know Yourself* (Third Edition). Burgess Publishing Company: Minneapolis, 1958.

Byrne, Renee, *Let's Talk About Stuttering*. George Allen: London, 1983.

Carlisle, Jock A., *Tangled Tongue: Living with a Stutter*. Addison Wesley Publishing Company, Inc.: Reading, MA, 1985.

Conture, Edward G., *Stuttering*. Prentice-Hall, Inc.: Englewood Cliffs, NJ, 1982.

Cooper, Eugene, B., *Personalized Fluency Control Therapy: An Integrated Behavior and Relationship Therapy for Stutterers*. Teaching Resources Corporation: Highham, MA, 1976.

*Counseling Stutterers*, Pub., No. 18. Speech Foundation of America: Memphis, TN, undated.

Dalton, Peggy, *Approaches to the Treatment of Stuttering*. Croom Helm: London, 1983.

Eisenson, John (Editor), *Stuttering, A Symposium*. Harper and Row: New York, 1958.

Fraser, Malcolm, *Self-Therapy for the Stutterer*, Pub. No. 12, Third Ed., Speech Foundation of America: Memphis, TN, 1978.

Gregory, Hugo H. (Editor), *Controversies about Stuttering Therapy*. University Park Press: Baltimore, 1979.

Gregory, Hugo H. (Editor), *Learning Theory and Stuttering Therapy*. Northwestern University Press: Evanston, IL, 1968.

Guitar, B., and Peters, T.J., *Stuttering: an Integration of Contemporary Therapies*. Pub. No. 16. Speech Foundation of America: Memphis, TN, 1980.

Hulit, Lloyd M., *Stuttering: In Perspective*. Charles C Thomas: Springfield, IL, 1985.

Hulit, Lloyd, *Stuttering Therapy*. Charles C Thomas: Springfield, IL, 1985.

Jacobson, Edward, *Progressive Relaxation*. University of Chicago Press: Chicago, 1938.

Jacobson, Edmund, *You Must Relax*. McGraw-Hill Book Co.: New York, 1957.

Jonas, Gerald, *Stuttering, the Disorder of Many Theories*. Farrar Straus and Giroux: New York, 1976.

Murphy, Albert T. and Ruth M. Fitz-Simons, *Stuttering and Personality Dynamics*. Ronald Press Company: New York, 1960.

Murray, Frederick, *A Stutterer's Story*. Interstate Printers and Publishers, Inc.: Danville, Illinois, 1980.

Peins, Maryanne (Editor), *Contemporary Approaches in Stuttering Therapy*. Little, Brown & Co.: Boston, 1984.

Preus, Alf, *Identifying Subgroups of Stutterers*. Universitet-forlaget: Oslo, Norway, 1981.

Rieber, R.W. (Editor), *The Problem of Stuttering*. Elsevier: New York, 1977.

Robinson, Frank B., *Introduction to Stuttering*. Prentice-Hall, Inc.: Englewood Cliffs, NJ, 1964.

Schwartz, Martin F., *Stuttering Solved*. J.B. Lippincot Company: Philadelphia, 1976.

Shames, George H. and Donald B. Egolf, *Operant Conditioning and the Management of Stuttering*. Prentice-Hall Inc.: Englewood Cliffs, NJ, 1976.

Shames, George H. and Cheri L. Florence, *Stutter-free Speech: A Goal for Therapy*. Charles E. Merrill Publishing Co.: Columbus, OH, 1980.

Sheehan, Joseph (Editor), *Stuttering: Research and Therapy*. Harper and Row: New York, 1970.

Silverman, Franklin H., *Relapse following Stuttering Therapy*. Academic Press, Inc.: San Diego, California, 1981.

St. Louis, Kenneth O., *The Atypical Stutterer*. Academic Press, Inc.: San Diego, California, 1986.

Starkweather, C. Woodruff, *Fluency and Stuttering*. Prentice-Hall, Inc.: Englewood Cliffs, NJ, 1987.

Starkweather, C. Woodruff, *Stuttering: Successes and Failures in Therapy*, Pub. No. 6. Speech Foundation of America: Memphis, TN, 1987.

Travis, Lee Edward, "The Unspeakable Feelings of People with Special Reference to Stuttering", *Handbook of Speech Pathology and Audiology*. Prentice-Hall: Englewood Cliffs, NJ, 1971.

Van Riper, Charles, *The Nature of Stuttering* (Second Edition). Prentice-Hall, Inc.: Englewood Cliffs, NJ, 1982.

Van Riper, Charles, *The Treatment of Stuttering*. Prentice-Hall, Inc.: Englewood Cliffs, NJ, 1973.

Weiss, Deso A., *Cluttering*. Prentice-Hall, Inc.: Englewood Cliffs, NJ, 1964.

Wells, G. Beverly, *Stuttering Treatment*. Prentice-Hall, Inc.: Englewood Cliffs, NJ, 1987.

Wingate, Marcel E., *Stuttering: Theory and Therapy*. Irvington Publishers, Inc.: New York, 1976.

# APPENDICES

# Appendix A

## THE NATURE OF STUTTERING ACCORDING TO LEOPOLD TREITEL

Morris Val Jones

*Studying German, I ran across an 1894 article written by a Berlin physician, Dr. Leopold Treitel, discussing the nature and phenomenology of stuttering. Amazingly, Dr. Treitel's article contains some current theories on the highly debated causes of this condition. Therefore, a partial translation will still inform modern speech correctionists. He wrote as follows:*

Stuttering is a nervous illness, characterized by tonic [vocal chord held closed] or clonic [vocal chord fluttered open and closed] spasms of certain groups of the speech muscles. These contractions can affect also the musculature of the larynx, palate, tongue and breathing mechanism, either singly or in groups. The spasms may extend to other neck or facial muscles, causing grimaces which may unwittingly provoke onlookers to laugh inappropriately. These movements are only 'with-movements,' as [are] gestures while speaking. These 'with-movements' often extend themselves to the arms... and legs. Gutzmann tells of the case of a man who before each attempt to speak first bent together and then sprang forward in order to finally bring forth a word. He was proclaimed deranged and brought to an asylum, where Herr Professor Westphal recognized his illness as stuttering.

Separately the phonatory spasms present very different pictures. Spasms of the breathing area may occur during inhalation as well as in exhalation. Before or in the middle of a word the stutterer must suddenly grasp for breath even though his supply of air is not exhausted or even diminished. These inhalations, which are caused by spasms of the diaphragm—Coen believed—enable the stutterer to take care of a defective air pressure.

I have refuted this contention, however, by my spirometrical examinations. These same spasms may occur during exhalation; they come suddenly and jerkingly at the beginning or in the middle of speech. It seems to me that exhalation spasms are more frequent than inhalation spasms. During the exhalation spasms no sound can be produced; during inhalation spasms sound is possible, but most stutterers sound more as if they are gagging. As Ssikorski reports, in both cases one can hear an "h" at the end of most tonic spasms so that, for example the word "Stottern" becomes "Sth-ottern" and the word "Tadel," becomes "Tah-ha-ha-hadel." In severe cases inhalation and exhalation spasms appear alternately.

The musculature of the larynx and the breathing mechanism is affected. Usually the closing mechanism rather than the opening mechanism is involved, and generally the picture changes according to whether the muscles are in tonic or clonic spasm. During a tonic spasm it is either impossible to phonate, or the vowel is prolonged abnormally. During the clonic spasm, the voice is repeated (bleating). The inability to produce a sound has misled several authors to look upon this as a special illness and call it by a particular name (spasmus glottidis phonatorius, dysphonia spastica); these cases are, however, nothing more than a special form of stuttering. If the front neck musculature is affected, then the head drops and the mouth is open, making a very comic [sic] sight.

During tonic spasms of the intrinsic speech musculature, the consonant is held a long time; during clonic spasms, it is often repeated, as, for example, "P---apa," or "P-p-p-p-p-papa." The spasms appear mainly during loud speaking and reading, less during whispering and seldom during singing. They are usually absent also if the patient speaks to himself or within a circle of friends. On the other hand, they can appear, for example, while telephoning. They tend to be strongest if the stutterer finds himself with a stranger, the more so the higher the stranger's social rank. [Editor's note: Also, the taller the stranger is.]

Research proves that there are psychic influences which produce speech spasms. Denhardt calls the illness a "psychose." Other skills—such as playing musical instruments, writing, and even walking—can be affected by psychic influences. The stutterer, with rare exceptions, is affected by anxiety felt in the pit of the stomach. Young children, however, tend to know nothing of this feeling. Of 180 children between the ages of 3 to 6 years, 24 (or 13%) spoke with interruptions accompanied by spasms in the speech musculature.

I believe I can show that these blocks result because [the child's mind directs its body to] begin to speak before the awkward speech organs [have received the complete message]. Especially if there are [physical?] articulatory defects or even only difficulty in the pronunciation of sounds, the child tries to begin to speak before he knows [how to say] what to he wants to say [, how to form the desired sounds.] It is also characteristic of this speech blocking that the children are somewhat delayed for their age in the formation of unusual or difficult speech sounds and they repeat familiar consonants—for example, *m, n, b, f,* etc. These children are rarely stutterers, but they can become so. Although interruptions of speech and quivering of the speech musculature occasionally occur in children, with the stutterer they are accompanied by a sometimes subconscious imaginary necessity to make certain sounds. How does this imagining develop? Among the several causes are a nervous basis and particular circumstances.

The nervousness is almost always inherited; rarely is it produced by a weakening illness. Deformity of the speech organs is not a predisposing cause; it can produce articulatory defects but not stuttering. If the stuttering stops after the removal of growths in the nasal pharynx, this is to be traced to the psychological influence of the operation [i.e., power of suggestion].

As far as the inheritance of stuttering is concerned, Gutzmann ascribes it no great role; and I can, so far as my research justifies, not ascribe it as great importance as Ssikorski and Denhardt have done. Ssikorski found that 31% of 359 stutterers were familial stutterers; Denhardt's figure [more than doubles this]. He declares to have found 1,545 of 1,994 stuttering cases, or 77.5%, traceable to heredity. [Yet] Coen has been able to establish only 11%, 36 hereditary influences among 335. [So] Heredity does [appear to] play a certain role in the onset of stuttering.

Stuttering may grow out of an illness. Herr Professor Mendel tells of the 15 year old Gustav B, who spoke faultlessly at the beginning of his nervous illness, Freidrich's disease. As the disease progressed, the speech became more and more difficult. At the time of my examination, he showed obvious signs of embarrassment; while speaking he blushed, lowered his eyes, and looked elsewhere. He experienced anxiety while talking with strangers, more so than while speaking with persons whom he knew. "With-movements" were very pronounced, consisting partly of spasmodic quivering of the face, of the neck and of the right arm, and partly of quivering of the lips during and after the speech. The pronunciation of a single sound — especially the lip sounds, *b, p, f, m,* — at the beginning of a sentence became extremely difficult. He delayed on them a long time while he pressed the lips tightly together; meanwhile, the beginning consonant was repeated. The same elongation was true with vowels. He was nevertheless capable of pronouncing all sounds correctly, except the ones which seemed to him especially difficult. He spoke more easily if one [first] pronounced for him. His brother, who was three years older and had the same illness, spoke strikingly slower, chopped the syllables off, and prolonged the beginning consonants longer than usual; but he spoke without anxiety and did not show symptoms of embarrassment, although he made use of some "with-movements" while speaking.

The first case shows how stuttering can develop on the basis of an organic illness. The older brother had almost the same speech defect as the younger, but he did not become a stutterer; that is, he lacked the anxiety feeling which leads to the resulting speech disorder. This may have been because he was older and already more calm or because he was less excitable. Thus, we see how stuttering may develop in children; namely, if it is [precipitated by] an hereditary nervousness. The speech defect in turn produces [more] anxiety, and this increased anxiety produces [more] speech defect; thus a vicious cycle develops for the stutterer. Later, the anxiety feeling produces the most conspicuous symptoms, [just] as in many illnesses a symptom endures long after the origin has disappeared, e.g., the running of the ears after scarlet fever. One must not, however, as Schrank has done, present the anxiety as the causative factor.

In most cases, the [child's consciousness of] his stuttering begins before he starts school. [Presumably, in 1894, this meant before broad exposure to children outside the family.] The parents themselves have made the child conscious of the errors and through threats or stern treatment produced in him that timidity which further completes the picture of the stutterer. [This could be heridatory or imitation if source is available.]

In many cases, however, the child first [encounters] speech difficulties when he starts school [or day care imitating the speech of a stutterering classmate. This] "psychic contamination," undoubtedly plays a great role in [the] increase [of stuttering]. Children imitate everything much more easily than adults, and therefore learn simply whatever is taught them [or they are exposed to] at school. But they learn the bad as well as the good; in fact, the former ever more easily than the latter. Even the younger children show this tendency to imitate; they cry as soon as a strange child cries.

One can also observe this involuntary imitation with adults; for example, when somebody starts coughing at a concert, many follow him. Still more obvious is psychic contamination in the case of nervous people; for example, when a hysterical girl has a convulsive attack, other women with similar dispositions in the same ward have attacks. [Editors note: Presumably, today at least, male patients can have similar attacks.]

The following case illustrates that the playing together of two children can be responsible for the onset of stuttering: Rosalie G., ten years old, daughter of a businessman, is not tainted by heredity. [Editor's note: Today this conclusion might be challenged: Just because none of her sisters or parents stutters does not exclude hereditary causes.] She has three [older] sisters, none of whom stutters. Her physical and mental development was normal, she proved in her bearing no abnormality; she got along well in school. In the fifth year of life she played for a long time together with a stuttering boy. Although she had spoken well until then, she soon began to stutter. The father believed sternness would set her free from the illness, but it became worse; as a result the girl stutters more at home than with strangers. The form of the stuttering is a tonic spasmodic one.

With error, defective endowment [intelligence] was taken for granted as the cause of stuttering; on the contrary, the stutterers are on the average more endowed than others, even though many times through their involuntary silence they give an impression of stupidity. One must be cautious in accepting the influence of known circumstances, which for the stutterer may be important. The personal information of the stutterers is often not entirely sound because they may self-diagnose the cause of their stuttering by [mere] assumption. Such circumstancial influences may be the days and seasons, temperature variations, and even changes of the moon. Many circumstances may, however, affect indirectly the intensity of the stuttering; for example, climate or locality changes may influence the frame of mind of the stutterer; in certain conditions he stutters somewhat more or less.

Gutzmann ascribes an exaggerated influence to second teething and puberty upon the onset of stuttering. There are very few cases in which one can trace the onset of stuttering directly to second teething. Stuttering which develops at puberty is not stuttering at all but hysterical speech interruptions. What frequently happens is that an earlier occurrence reappears or is reinforced. The great psychical sensitivity of the time of puberty develops in the individual a conscious shyness of the feminine sex, which makes his voice uncertain, and his heart beat harder. The same thing may happen when he speaks to strangers. For example, Schulthess reports of himself that in his 15th year he stuttered for a certain time, but only if the word began with a "d"; after a few months the evil [sic] stopped of itself. One must also take into consideration that during this time examinations fall or the apprentice period begins. It would be, therefore, often questionable whether these happenings or puberty is guilty of the onset of stuttering. Moreover, stuttering decreases after puberty. The calm and self-possession of maturity give the psychic influences less importance than the impressionable spirit of adolescence. The diminution with age is to be assumed a proof of the psychic nature of these troubles. Even though it is not authoritative, the following table presented by Denhardt is very clear. Of the cases which he handled, the stutterers stand:

| Age 6–8 | 49 |
|---|---|
| 9–12 | 323 |
| 13–15 | 336 |
| 16–20 | 631 |
| 21–25 | 549 |
| 26–30 | 207 |
| 31–40 | 133 |
| 41–50 | 48 |
| 51–60 | 14 |
| 62 | 1 |

These figures are not conclusive, as they give only the ages of cases which Denhardt has handled and not the average ages of stutterers; but they are doubtless proportional [Editor's note: assuming randomized sample, etc.]. I have, for example, had more children than adults in my practice. The oldest stutterer who entrusted himself to me was 68 years old. [which just may mean that adult stutterers did not come in for therapy, at least not to Treitel.]

Stuttering may be caused by an injury—such as a fall, blow or concussion—or a violent fright. Even in cases of injury, fright may have significance for the onset of stuttering. But one may, as Coen has done, overrate the significance of these occasional causes. One must not always take at face value the reports of parents in these cases. Many times the parents assign one of those events as the cause, but upon closer examination most of them state that the stuttering [had been] present since an earlier age. [In order to prescribe the correct treatment, one must certainly establish whether the stuttering began after an infectious disease, such as measles, diphtheria, scarlet fever, typhus, or influenza. [Without a prior disease, the cause could be entirely psychological.]

Speech disorders are found more among the masculine than the feminine sex. One cannot trace these distinctions to physical differences, as Gutzmann has done. The distinction is more likely psychological. As we cannot make clear why girls on the average speak earlier than boys, so we cannot make clear why stuttering is less frequent among girls. While Coen found only 10% feminine stutterers, Denhardt's exhaustive study of 820,000 children found the female:male proportion was approximately 1:2.5 [29% female]. Similar results are reported by Gutzmann.

## Author's Comment

Amazingly, the majority of Dr. Treitel's positions *remain* viable after nearly a century of intensive research with much more refined techniques than those available to him and his colleagues. Members of the American Speech, Language, and Hearing Association have conducted thousands of studies in the past fifty years which have merely confirmed his statements. Modern experts on stuttering differ significantly from his conclusions in only two instances, maintaining that:

(1) imitation does not lead to the onset of stuttering, and
(2) second teething is not a possible cause of stuttering.

On this second point, however, Dr. Treitel had indicated that stuttering had probably occurred before puberty and that a diagnosis of stuttering in the teen years was likely related to recurrence.

# Appendix B

## SPEECH FOUNDATION OF AMERICA

A Non-Profit Organization
P.O. Box 11749
Memphis, TN 38111

Also producer of films and videotapes on stuttering

## Publications on Stuttering

*Please add per order*
*Handling Charge: Domestic $1.00, International $2.00*

No. 1—On *Stuttering* and Its Treatment, 56 pp., 1961—$.50
Published in the interest of making available to speech therapists and other interested parties, the agreements reached by a group of leading authorities concerning the methods to be used in helping to relieve the adult stutterer of his problem.

No. 2—*Stuttering* Words, revised, 48 pp., 1961—$.50.
An authoritative glossary of the meanings of the words and terms associated with the field of stuttering.

No. 3—*Stuttering.* Its Prevention, 64 pp., 1962—$.50.
For parents who do not want their children to stutter, especially for those parents of very young children who think they have reason to be concerned about their child's speech.

No. 4—*Stuttering.* Treatment of the Young Stutterer in the School, 64 pp., 1964—$.50.
Discussing problems encountered by the speech clinician working with stutterers in school. Answering questions asked by school clinicians about working therapy with the young stutterer.

No. 5—*Stuttering.* Training the Therapist. 96 pp., 1966—$.50.
An outline of a suggested course of study to be used in training speech pathology students how to cope with the baffling problems encountered in working with the stutterer.

No. 6—*Stuttering.* Successes and Failures in Therapy, 148 pp., 1968—$1.50.
Case histories of successes and failures in the treatment of stuttering by nine

leading speech pathologists describing the procedures and techniques used in each case and the results attained.

**No. 7—*Stuttering*. Conditioning in Stuttering Therapy (Applications and Limitations), 180 pp., 1970—$1.50.**

Exploring the conditioning approach to the treatment of stuttering with articles advocating its use and criticism of its desirability together with a summary of conference discussions and a glossary of conditioning terms.

**No. 8—*Stuttering*. An Account of Intensive Demonstration Therapy. 124 pp., 1971—$1.50.**

Report of a therapy project in which three master clinicians work with three stutterers intensively for a period of five weeks under the observation of fifteen experienced speech pathologists.

**No. 9—To the *Stutterer,* 116 pp., 1972—$1.50.**

Practical advice written by twenty-four men and women speech pathologists who have been stutterers, telling what helped them and advising what they believe will help the stutterer control the difficulty.

**No. 10—Therapy for *Stutterers,* 120 pp., 1974—$1.50.**

This book outlines a program for speech clinicians working with adult or older adolescent stutterers. Written by speech pathologists who have specialized in stuttering.

**No. 11—If Your Child *Stutters*. A Guide for Parents (Revised), 48 pp., 1988—$1.00.**

An authoritative and understandable book for parents. Contains examples of what to do to help young stutterers three to six years of age. Can be used as a supplement to clinical conference advice.

**No. 12—Self-Therapy for the *Stutterer:* One Approach (Sixth Edition), 184 pp., 1987—$2.50.**

Written for the adult who is unable to take advantage of clinical treatment— and outlines a self-therapy program which describes what the stutterer can and should do to tackle the problem and control the stuttering.

**No. 13—Treating the School Age *Stutterer*. A Guide for Clinicians, 112 pp., undated—$1.50.**

Describes how a clinician can work effectively with young stutterers. Written by a public school clinician who works exclusively with stutterers and who was trained as a stuttering specialist.

**No. 14—Si Su Hijo *Tartamudea:* Una Guia Para Los Padres—Spanish Translation of No. 11, "If Your Child Stutters: A Guide for Parents," 48 pp.—$1.00.**

**No. 15—*Stuttering:* An Integration of Contemporary Therapies, 80 pp.—$1.50.**

Explains how speech clinicians can combine the different but most commonly used treatment procedures to get effective results when working with stutterers of all ages.

**No. 16—Mon Enfant *Begnie-t-il?* Un Guide pour les Parents—French translation of No. 11, "If Your Child Stutters: A Guide for Parents," 44 pp.—$1.00.**

**No. 17—Counseling *Stutterers,* 80 pp., undated—$1.50.**
This book helps the clinician have a better understanding of the counseling aspect of therapy and suggests ways to use it effectively.

**No. 18—*Stuttering* Therapy: Transfer and Maintenance, 112 pp.—$1.50**
Discusses in depth the crucial role of transfer and maintenance and how they may be used to promote long lasting therapy results.

**No. 19—*Stuttering* Therapy: Prevention and Intervention with Children, (Edited by Hugo H. Gregory) 152 pp.—$1.50**
An in-depth discussion of the most recent procedures used in the prevention of stuttering and early intervention with children.

**No. 20—Do You *Stutter,* A Guide for Teens, 80 pp.—$1.00**
The first book written specifically for teen-agers outlines unique problems faced by the stuttering teen in dealing with parents, school and friends, and how to handle them successfully.

# Appendix C

## FLUENCY CHECKLIST

Below you will find a list of situations with which you may be familiar. For each situation, circle either 1—Always, 2—Most of the Time, 3—Sometimes, 4—Hardly Ever, or 5—Never. Answer only those items which apply to you. We are interested in knowing how fluent you are in various situations.

FLUENT SPEECH

|  | Always | Most of the Time | Sometimes | Hardly Ever | Never |
|---|---|---|---|---|---|
| 1. Talking on the telephone | 1 | 2 | 3 | 4 | 5 |
| 2. Talking to a stranger | 1 | 2 | 3 | 4 | 5 |
| 3. Giving your name | 1 | 2 | 3 | 4 | 5 |
| 4. Talking with a young child | 1 | 2 | 3 | 4 | 5 |
| 5. Placing an order in a restaurant | 1 | 2 | 3 | 4 | 5 |
| 6. Talking to an animal | 1 | 2 | 3 | 4 | 5 |
| 7. Talking with a close friend | 1 | 2 | 3 | 4 | 5 |
| 8. Arguing with parents | 1 | 2 | 3 | 4 | 5 |
| 9. Talking during casual conversation | 1 | 2 | 3 | 4 | 5 |
| 10. Responding to criticism | 1 | 2 | 3 | 4 | 5 |
| 11. Meeting someone for the first time | 1 | 2 | 3 | 4 | 5 |
| 12. Saying hello | 1 | 2 | 3 | 4 | 5 |
| 13. Reading aloud | 1 | 2 | 3 | 4 | 5 |
| 14. Answering a specific question | 1 | 2 | 3 | 4 | 5 |
| 15. Asking for information | 1 | 2 | 3 | 4 | 5 |
| 16. Being interviewed for a job | 1 | 2 | 3 | 4 | 5 |
| 17. Arguing a point | 1 | 2 | 3 | 4 | 5 |
| 18. Giving directions | 1 | 2 | 3 | 4 | 5 |
| 19. Talking when "high" | 1 | 2 | 3 | 4 | 5 |
| 20. Talking when trying to make a good impression | 1 | 2 | 3 | 4 | 5 |
| 21. Talking when happy | 1 | 2 | 3 | 4 | 5 |
| 22. Talking when depressed | 1 | 2 | 3 | 4 | 5 |
| 23. Speaking with one person | 1 | 2 | 3 | 4 | 5 |
| 24. Speaking with 2-3 people | 1 | 2 | 3 | 4 | 5 |
| 25. Speaking with 4-10 people | 1 | 2 | 3 | 4 | 5 |
| 26. Speaking with more than 10 people | 1 | 2 | 3 | 4 | 5 |
| 27. Apologizing | 1 | 2 | 3 | 4 | 5 |

| | | | | | |
|---|---|---|---|---|---|
| 28. Speaking when angry | 1 | 2 | 3 | 4 | 5 |
| 29. Speaking with a member of the opposite sex | 1 | 2 | 3 | 4 | 5 |
| 30. Speaking with someone you believe has a higher social or economic status than you | 1 | 2 | 3 | 4 | 5 |
| 31. Speaking with someone you believe has a lower social or economic status than you | 1 | 2 | 3 | 4 | 5 |
| 32. Speaking with an older person | 1 | 2 | 3 | 4 | 5 |
| 33. Speaking with a younger person | 1 | 2 | 3 | 4 | 5 |
| 34. Speaking with an aggressive person | 1 | 2 | 3 | 4 | 5 |
| 35. Speaking with a passive person | 1 | 2 | 3 | 4 | 5 |
| 36. Speaking with your boss or supervisor | 1 | 2 | 3 | 4 | 5 |
| 37. Speaking with coworkers | 1 | 2 | 3 | 4 | 5 |
| 38. Speaking with someone you supervise | 1 | 2 | 3 | 4 | 5 |
| 39. Buying something in a store | 1 | 2 | 3 | 4 | 5 |
| 40. Speaking when exhausted | 1 | 2 | 3 | 4 | 5 |

Total Number (Add the number of circles in each category) _____ _____ _____ _____ _____

Total Scores (Add the scores in each category) _____ _____ _____ _____ _____

Grand Total (Add the Total Scores) _____

Mean (Divide Grand Total by sum of Total Number scores) _____

Mode Score (Category above that had the greatest Total Number) _____

jg

# Appendix D

## LETTERS

The following letters are representative of those written by confirmed stutterers.

**A Social Worker From Cedar Falls, Iowa Writes:**

May 30, 1987

Dr. Val Jones
Department of Speech and Audiology
California State University
Sacramento, California 95819

Dear Dr. Jones:

I'm writing this in response to the NSP's April Notes insert. I've been a social worker for the last 15 years and have been plagued about every five years with stuttering bad enough to undermine communication skills and self-confidence. For the majority of the time I'm a "closet stutterer," capable to disguising and concealing—some of my close friends have not consciously recognized that I stutter until we've talked about it.

Anyway, approximately two years ago I began in therapy again through the University of Northern Iowa's Speech and Hearing Clinic (prior to that, at approximate five year intervals, I'd received therapy to slow down my rate of speech and at another time had used self-hypnosis tapes, both of them seemingly "worked", at least for several years). Because my stuttering is slight rather than severe (even though it feels just as terrifying), we've worked on pull outs, cancellations (both of which I detested but probably were essential—at least they made me really appreciate the preparatory sets) and preparatory sets. For me, the "prep sets" have been wonderful—I can scan ahead into the next few words and ease into the troublesome ones. Needless to say, I can't use them all of the time; if I'm rushing myself, sick, or under stress it takes extra energy to do this and sometimes I can't. But, the "prep sets" have been a life-saver for me. In combination with the supportive staff and their philosophy that you've got to work on it daily, the realization that you're still going to slip up sometimes makes it a lot easier to handle. I know that I'm still going to have about five below average days every month but at least now I have the tools to work with (my tennis isn't too hot then, either)!

I also think that we, as a group, tend to be extremely self-critical and fail to make the same allowances for ourselves that we'd make for others.

Good luck with your book.

Sincerely,

L.L.

**A Housewife From San Bruno, California Writes:**

April 27, 1987

Dear Sir,

I read in the NSP newsletter, "Letting Go," that you are asking for information on the fluent experiences of stutterers. I am a 47-year-old housewife with five children, and I have stuttered as long as I can remember, in varying degrees of severity. I have come to the conclusion that, as stuttering is primarily a physiological problem, I have to keep myself in as healthy a physical and emotional state as possible, in order to achieve fluency. For instance, the less "junk food," caffeine, sugar, and salt I absorb, the better my speech. These products do have an influence on our brains and physical well-being. After a complete physical check-up, I was found to have an iron-deficiency anemia, also a B-12 deficiency, as I am unable to absorb vitamin B-12 orally and have to have monthly shots of the vitamin. I wonder how many others have vitamin deficiencies which can only be diagnosed by a physician, and whose stuttering is affected by it.

Also, exercise plays a very important role. Another method of achieving fluency is "imaging," which means to imagine oneself in a situation, speaking fluently. This is really phenomenal, as it really words so easily! The latest findings on the workings of the brain prove that just thinking about an action will provoke the physical response of that action.

The third, and final, means of attaining fluency is simply that "practice makes perfect." Just simply living long enough to do the feared action over and over again, e.g., calling the doctor; answering the phone, will provide a lessening anxiety each successive time, and the less the anxiety, the less the stuttering.

The basis for my fluency achieved through good health is the therapy I had with Dr. Leo Sack, of South San Francisco. It included "imagery" and the emphasis on good health and exercise, although I would emphasize a physical examination which shows more information on vitamin deficiency that the "vitamin expert" that Dr. Sack referred me to. The *relaxation* therapy was very important also.

In conclusion, my fluency is the result of treatment for my iron and vitamin B12 deficiencies, and maintaining a healthy lifestyle; imagery; and lessening anxiety of a feared experience by doing it until it becomes non-anxiety producing. The only time I have experienced difficulty in speaking recently has been at the monthly menstrual cycle, when hormones go what can only be described as crazy and unpredictable. That, too, can only be cured by growing older!

Good luck, and hope to hear about some other "cures" in your book.

Sincerely,

B.C.L.

P.S. All of the above procedures result, hopefully in a more positive, relaxed self-image, which is crucial in fluent speaking. I am of the minority of stutterers who do *not* force myself into a speaking situation when I *know* that I am not feeling well enough to have some control, much as I would not force an epileptic in the midst of a seizure to do what is impossible at that time.

I have learned enough about my *own* speech to know what works for me, and that includes pausing before a block and recognizing that two conflicting thoughts or words in my mind at the same time will produce a block, as if my brain cannot choose which word or idea to pursue, so therefore is *unable* to make a choice without blocking.

# Appendix E

## PROFESSIONAL JOURNALS

Many professional journals contain articles about stuttering. Among those which emphasize disfluency are the following:

*American Journal of Psychotherapy*
*Journal of Abnormal Psychology*
*Journal of Communication Disorders*
*Journal of Fluency Disorders*
*Journal of Experimental Analysis of Behavior*
*Journal of Speech and Hearing Disorders*
*Journal of Speech and Hearing Research*
*Language, Speech and Hearing Services in Schools*
*Perception and Motor Skills*

These journals are probably not available in the public libraries. University libraries, especially those which service programs in speech pathology, usually subscribe to the above-listed journals. In addition, many other journals have occasional articles about disfluency.

Appendix—F

## THE NATIONAL STUTTERING PROJECT

1269 Seventh Avenue
San Francisco, California 94122
415-566-5324

Welcome to the **National Stuttering Project.** For over 10 years, we have been meeting the needs of children and adults who stutter. There are three million of them in the United States, and the NSP wants to get our message of hope to all of them.

The NSP is a non-profit organization with 2,500 members nationwide. Our activities are divided into these basic areas:

• We provide information on all aspects of stuttering to people who stutter as well as to their friends and relatives, and to the general public.

• We serve as a referral service for those people seeking professional help. And through our self-help chapter meetings and workshops, we provide a safe, supportive environment where people who stutter can learn to communicate more effectively.

• Most importantly, we let people know that **if they are dealing with a stuttering problem, they do not have to do it alone.** Most of our members are those who, themselves, deal with a stuttering problem.


## What the NSP Can Do For You


**FIRST OF ALL,** let us tell you what the NSP is **not** going to do for you.

We have **no** new breathing technique or miracle diet which is going to give you the breakthrough you may have been waiting for.

We are **not** in the business of speech therapy. We are not professionals who will guide you through a program of some kind.

**We do offer you an opportunity to help yourself and others, too.** We can help you discover some of the factors that contribute to your stuttering. And we can provide the environment and the information you need to look past your stuttering to discover who **you** are.

Most of us have been so aware of how we speak that we tend to filter our life experiences through the framework of "being a stutterer." Stuttering seems to color everything we do. Consequently, we become blind to our other qualities and attributes.

At NSP chapter meetings, workshops, and other functions, we don't care whether you stutter or not; in fact, it's the norm. You'll find that this will take the pressure off your having to speak "correctly" and allow you to focus your attention on other things you are doing and being.

The NSP will allow you to develop your abilities on a number of different fronts. In many cases, this will allow you to express yourself with greater ease and fluency. You will be surprised how much of the pressure you're under will be relieved when stuttering is not something you have to hide from the world. Perhaps stuttering has seemed such a burden for you in the past because you have had to carry it alone. **With the NSP, stuttering will lose much of its sting because you do not have to feel different any more.**

**The NSP is designed to be fun.** Involvement with us is not one of those grit-your-teeth-and-bear-it experiences, but an opportunity for self-discovery and a chance to let yourself soar. If you allow it, the National Stuttering Project will help you . . .

**Have more fun while speaking.** If you are like most people, speaking was always a matter of survival . . . a question of "Can I get through it this time?" No wonder we've avoided speaking situations.

In the NSP you'll discover a direct correlation between freer speech and the ability to have fun while talking. Perhaps this is because when you are having fun, you're pleasing yourself rather than someone else. In the supportive environment of the NSP chapter meetings and workshops, and through the information provided in our publications, you can discover how to loosen up, be more yourself, and become more grounded. If you've never known what it is to have fun as a speaker, this can be a real breakthrough.

**Improve your ability to relate to others.** It is hard to be comfortable with others if you experience yourself as strange or different. Most of us have been "in the closet" regarding our stuttering. We've tried to hide it, sometimes at great cost to ourselves. We have never shared our feelings about our stuttering with other people. We've tended to either deny that the stuttering is there, or we have tried to wish it away. In other words, we have pretended to be someone we are not. In struggling to be "normal," we've continued to reinforce our own self image as being different. And this helps create a barrier between ourselves and those we come into contact with.

The fact is, we are very much like everybody else. We have simply blown up one of our differences way out of proportion. We have the opportunity to share our "unique" experiences . . . and hear or read about the experiences of others . . . we find out that we're not so unusual after all. We can learn that people will accept us even if we haven't attained total fluency.

**In fact, the rule seems to be: your listener will be as comfortable about your stuttering as you are.**

**Seeing things as they really are.** To bring about change, you first have to stop pretending and accept where you are. If you want to change how you speak, you must first get clear about the way you speak . . . about what you do and how you feel. (Hearing the experience of others can help in this.) Then you can begin to understand the things that block you from being more self-expressive.

The NSP can help you discover that accepting where you are **right now** is totally okay.

**Assist others.** Anyone who stutters would admit that living with the problem has taught them things about life and about themselves. In the NSP you will have a chance to share what you've learned with others to help them grow. In doing so, you will discover your own secret resources, and how much you already know about the problem of stuttering.

You will come to appreciate that the NSP is not a one-way street. We are not here to just help you. You can take pride in helping others by your involvement with us.

**Practice what you are learning in speech therapy.** Although we, ourselves, do not conduct speech therapy, we are still all for it. Many members of the NSP have taken extensive speech therapy or are in therapy now. You can learn and accomplish things through the facilitation of a speech therapist that we cannot deal with in our bi-weekly meetings or publications. But we can be an invaluable adjunct to any therapy program.

The NSP will assist those of you who are looking for a good speech therapy program if that is your interest. We have more contacts in this area than any other group.

Furthermore, the NSP can be the perfect training ground to practice what you are learning in a speech therapy program with people that understand what you are trying to accomplish and how difficult it is. We can help you generalize your clinical success to real life situations. And we can assist you in solidifying your gains.

## NSP Self-Help Chapters

The National Stuttering Project operates 55 self-help groups around the United States.

These meetings give you a chance to share your experience with others, to assume responsibility for your own growth, and to foster the growth of others.

We could fill up many pages with the success stories that have come out of these meetings. The meetings will change your life if you give them a chance.

Check with us to see whether there is an NSP chapter near you. If there is not, we can put you in contact with other NSP members near you; together, perhaps, you can get one going. We have a lengthy guide that explains just how to do this.

## "Letting Go"

The next best thing to being at a chapter meeting is reading what members share in our monthly newsletter, "Letting Go."

Every month, "Letting Go" will remind you that you are not alone, that others feel what you feel, do what you do, think what you think.

"Letting Go" will make you laugh and cry, but most of all it will make you feel good.

## NSP Brochures

The National Stuttering Project puts out the following brochures. They are available for 50 cents each.

- To My Friends Who Stutter: Some Considerations
- A Brochure for Parents of Children Who Stutter
- What the Teacher Can Do to Help the Child Who Stutters
- A Person's Journey Through Stuttering
- Shopping for a Speech Pathologist
- Non-Avoidance: The Wisdom of Joseph Sheehan, Ph.D.

## NSP Tapes

**NSP Tape Series**
*(All tapes are $8):*

- The Parents Tape
- A Presentation of the NSP
- A Typical NSP Chapter Meeting
- The Precision Fluency Shaping Program
- The NSP Stories Tape
- A Message for Teenagers
- A Talk by Fred Murray
- The School Clinician Tape
- A Stuttering Demonstration
- Stuttering, 1957

# National Stuttering Project
# (NSP)

Kay Robison
Supervisor of Speech Therapy
Sacramento City Schools, California

The National Stuttering Project (NSP) was founded in 1977 by Bob Goldman and Michael Sugarman in San Francisco.

It is not a treatment strategy, nor is it in the business of providing therapy.

Mrs. Robison presented this material on the NSP as a panel member at the workshop "Stuttering Update" on April 5, 1983, at California State University, Sacramento sponsored by the CSUC Department of Speech Pathology and Audiology.

The NSP is a national organization, with chapters throughout the country. It publishes a monthly newsletter. This newsletter often becomes a forum about different kinds of therapy, whether traditional or new ones on the horizon. It also contains a lot of information about recent publications in the area of stuttering, really good information for anyone interested in the field. The NSP also provides information about where speech pathologists are in the country that do work with stuttering.

The NSP distributes pamphlets and brochures that contain information about stuttering; these are written for parents, teachers, and people in the community. NSP nationally also provides information to the media, so that national magazines and television spot announcements can heighten awareness about the knowledge pertaining to stuttering. The heart, or the core of NSP, is the local chapter meeting.

What is accomplished in the local meetings? In the first place, the meetings are fun. A very important part of NSP is to build into the experience some enjoyment and fun. The meetings are usually held twice a month. They are free. They are open to all persons who stutter. They are open to family members, friends, and professionals working with stutterers. The chapter meetings focus on growth in three different areas: speaking, personal awareness, and responsibility. Responsibility is learned at the chapter meeting because the meetings are facilitated by the participants. In other words, the stutterers, themselves, facilitate, along with family members or who ever else is there. But there is no one authority figure who comes in and takes charge of the meeting. The members themselves make NSP work. This is really helpful because many stutterers may feel that they are helpless. Because of their disorder, they often are searching for some authority to hand them a cure. We all know that isn't going to happen.

If they are going to make improvement influency they must take responsibility for themselves. This is something that NSP stresses, and really endeavors to make the participants realize, because at the meetings, everyone's opinions and ideas are equal. It does not matter whether one is a speech pathologist with a Ph.D. or a high school senior who still has a lot of disfluencies, their ideas on the causes or the cures of stuttering are equally worthy of presentation. So there is no one at the meetings to take responsibility; it is up to each member of the chapter.

The members come together to share what's been going on in their lives, and in their heads, since the last meeting. While meetings do provide a free space for persons who stutter or any of the participants, there is no guarantee that this is necessarily a comfortable experience. It is true that the meeting provides a protective environment, but NSP also stresses the fact that stutterers must be willing to take the risks to make changes.

So the chapter meetings actually become a different sort of experience for different people. For some stutterers, this might be an entry level experience. The stutterer might be a person who has had some therapy as a child, and perhaps that was not even a very pleasant experience, but has not had any additional therapy since. The NSP would be a beginning step, and during the sharing sessions he may hear other persons talking about therapy groups, and this person, this beginning person, might go into some of these types of formal therapy.

Also NSP can provide a carry-over experience for the person who is in therapy. Whatever techniques they are practicing, at the NSP meetings, can be utilized in the outside world. Meetings can also provide experience for the person who stuttered at one time and is now cured. At least these persons have achieved the level of fluency where they feel very comfortable and feel they can keep [maintain] the rest of their lives. These persons find at the meetings a chance to go over what caused the stuttering, or what it meant in their lives.

The chapter meetings provide a place where people can share these feelings and ideas. One way meetings facilitate the ability to talk about these very personal experiences, is that we do have one ironclad rule in our chapter, and that is that no participant tells another one what they should or shouldn't be doing. Each participant speaks from his or her own experience, and that makes the meeting a place there it is safe to express what has been happening because no one is going to be criticizing or giving advice. So there is no need to build up defenses.

For example, an adult stutterer might have it in his head that his stuttering was caused by his father who beat him behind the woodshed when he was 3 years old, or something of that sort. In other words, this could be an adult stutterer who is into a lot of blame. He has been carrying this blame around. That stutterer might hear another participant who is the mother of a young child who is stuttering. He can hear this mother say that it tears her heart to hear her child block so that she can't get the word out. So the other adult stutterer begins to realize that stuttering in his family was an interactional kind of process.

The speech pathologist in the group may hear another stutterer talk about how embarassing it was for him as a child, when he was in school, and they would announce over the loud speaker that it was time for him to go to speech class. That speech pathologist can hear that without feeling that she is being criticized for what she does, but maybe she will become a little more sensitive about how our clients do feel. Or the stutterers in the group may hear the speech pathologist talk about how she has problems getting up in front of a group. Having speaking fears is a universal feeling and the stutterers can realize that they are not some unique creature different from everybody else. So these are the kinds of things that go on during the sharing part of the meeting.

After this first half of the meeting, we take a coffee break, have refreshments, and just do some socializing. And then we come back to the fun part. And I think this is something rather unique to NSP. We do extemporaneous speaking. All participants. Stutterers, whoever else is there, and everyone picks out a topic. These topics are not necessarily about stuttering, but perhaps about Mrs. Reagan, or what you would order in a restaurant if money were no barrier, or where you would like to go for a vacation.

I wish you could hear some of the unique topics dreamed up at these meetings. The topics are thrown into a hat, and participants each pick one, and can talk for two minutes or two seconds, whatever. But after they are through talking, a couple of really important things take place. First of all, the speakers reflect on how they felt while they were speaking. This does a couple of really important things. It clears the air of any negative feeling that might have happened while the person was speaking. Then, too, the speakers can talk about what they are proud of and what felt good while they were talking. When the speakers are through with the speeches and their reflections about what they felt, the persons in the group give positive feedback, nothing negative, for example, "Gee, I really enjoyed it, and you had terrific eye contact while you were talking," etc. or "your voice sounded so alive while you were talking," and "I could just picture what you were talking about." As a person participates in many of these NSP meetings, I can tell you that they really feel good to hear that praise. Of course, there is a part of your brain that intellectualizes that these are the rules. Of course, the participants are following the rules to share things that are good only, but on an emotional level, the gut level, it really feels good to hear that praise.

---

According to John Ahlbach, Executive Director, the National Stuttering Project now has 2500 members. Memberships come from every state, and there are 55 local chapters. The highlight of the year has been the annual national convention; the Fourth Annual Convention was held on the campus of the California State University, San Francisco, in August, 1987. Information about the organization and membership applications are available by writing to 1269 Seventh Avenue, San Francisco, CA 94422.

# Testimonials

I can never repay the NSP for all the motivation and pride it has given me! Now, for the first time, I am feeling good about myself. I can do whatever I want—I'm OK!

*Jon Hawthorne*
*Baskin, Louisiana*

*Letting Go* continues to rank with my most absorbing reading.

*Oliver Bloodstein, Ph.D.*
*Brooklyn College, City University of New York*

As a speech/language pathologist, I am often faced with the task of understanding and sympathizing with the person who stutters . . . I feel your publication, *Letting Go,* is one of great value and interest to speech pathologists. We need to hear as many insights into the problem as possible.

*Deborah Partridge*
*Steinbach, Manitoba*

I read over each copy of *Letting Go* often, especially when I am having a bad day. Knowing I am not alone helps a great deal.

*Jim Heinz*
*Waukesha, Wisconsin*

The most beautiful thing that happened, however, was that after the meeting, when people were free to leave, they chose instead to stay and have another cup of coffee and talk—and talk—and talk! If they had had their choice, I believe they might have stayed through to the next meeting.

*Linda Holt (On the first meeting of Self Help Group in Buffalo.)*

When I first sent off my NSP membership, I was very afraid of being exposed so I gave my initials, M.J. Stocker. After reading the back issues of *Letting Go* you sent me, I realized I was trying to HIDE . . . I am Martha Stocker and I stutter.

*Martha Jane Stocker*
*Louisville, Kentucky*

I have needed you for a long time. Now that I have found the NSP, I don't believe I can ever let you go.

*Kay Shipton*
*Waukegan, Illinois*

When I would get depressed in the past about my stuttering, I would ask, "Why me?" Now I ask myself, "What can I do in the NSP to help other people who stutter.

*Claire Byrne*
*Los Angeles, California*

I have heard many good things about the National Stuttering Project.

*Annie Glenn*

I have to read each issue of *Letting Go* for the first time in private. A 58-year-old man is not supposed to cry, but some of the letters touch a part of me that triggers the tears.

*Revel Vines*
*Denver, Colorado*

After reading of other people's problems and the various professional opinions of what causes stuttering, I have been able to work on my problem tremendously.

*James Ford*
*Ray Brook, New York*

Keep up the good work. NSP is a lifeline which is greatly needed.

*Mike Thompson*
*Richmond, Virginia*

After just re-reading several issues of Letting Go, my mind is filled with similar experiences. Because I have "been there," I want so much to reach out my hand and pull each person that still lets stuttering shackle their lives past that final barrier—themselves.

*Bill Mahler*
*Fenton, Michigan*

I was delighted to become a member of the NSP and was impressed by the quantity and quality of your publications.

*Einer Boberg, Ph.D.*
*University of Alberta*

It's a wonderful feeling to know that we who stutter have a self-help group. Where have you been all my life? You do everything in such a warm, accepting and enthusiastic manner.

*Douglas Grote*
*Fanwood, New Jersey*

It is nice to see that someone notices that stuttering is worth forming a national organization about. This is very serious business. We need help. It really hurt not being able to express things the way you really want to. Bravo for the NSP!!

*Michael Busse*
*Mahwah, New Jersey*

I am very impressed! My immediate reaction is that everything you do is "right."

*Nancy Cohen*
*Reston, Virginia*

## THE SUCCESSFUL LIVING SERIES
## OF GUIDED RELAXATION TAPES

DAVID LEE

- Relax Your Way to a Better Life
- Expand the Power of Your Mind
- Achieve Your Goals Easily & Safely With Self-Hypnosis

*Light Shines in the Peaceful Mind*

It has been known since earliest times that guided relaxation is an extremely effective tool for self-improvement. Self-hypnosis tapes offer an easy and effective way to achieve goals through the process of relaxation learning. The hypnosis tape guides you safely into a calm, restful state in which your mind and body are completely relaxed. Then, gentle, positive suggestions allow your subconscious mind to accept the benefits that will occur through achieving your desired goal. Your subconscious mind is then able to work in harmony with your conscious mind to bring about the desired results. You come out of your relaxed state easily, whenever you want to, feeling alert and refreshed and you continue to feel good for many hours.

### Enjoy Relaxation Often While
### You Expand Your Potential

Guided relaxation tapes are a safe and effective way to transform your life. They are most effective when played frequently. The tapes can be used day or night, whenever a few minutes are available for relaxation. They can be played on first awakening in the morning or last thing at night. At night they are a wonderfully effective way to get to sleep if insominia is a problem. An inexpensive earplug or headset allows the tapes to be played at any time without disturbing others. **Since the tapes may cause drowsiness while being played, do not listen to hypnosis tapes while driving.**

## Relax as Your Therapist Guides You
## Towards Achievement of Your Goals

David Lee has used guided relaxation hypnotherapy for many years in his psychotherapy practice. He is a licensed Marriage, Family and Child Counselor and is also certified by the State of California to use hypnosis. David Lee has studied hypnosis extensively and has had instruction from many masters including Milton Erickson. He has conducted workshops in hypnotherapy and is Director of the Center for Counseling in Santa Monica, California. He also has a doctorate in engineering and has taught both engineering and psychology at the University of Southern California. He is a consultant to several aerospace companies and is also involved in a number of business ventures.

Mindstar Tapes
2210 Wilshire Boulevard
Suite 604
Santa Monica, California 90403

# Appendix H

## EXAMPLES OF MASTERS' THESES
## FROM CALIFORNIA STATE UNIVERSITY, SACRAMENTO
## ON SELECTED ASPECTS OF STUTTERING

**Becker, Stephanie Kay, Measurement and Comparison on Interaural Phase Disparity in Stutterers and Normal Speakers, 1977.**

The purpose of this study was to replicate the experiment performed by Stromsta (1972) in which he utilized the process of cancellation to compare interaural phase differences in stutterers and normal speakers. Accordingly, the experimental subjects in this study cancelled a bone-conducted tone by appropriate phase and amplitude adjustments of bilateral air-conducted tones at each of six frequencies. The time shift between the bilateral air-conducted signals at the point of cancellation served as the critarion measure of interaural phase disparity. In Experiment 1, three normal speakers participated in six trials in order to estimate the difficulties involved in the procedure. In Experiment 2, the procedure was used with seven stutterers over a two-trial period for comparison with Stromsta's study.

Within the limits of the present study, the following conclusions are warranted:

1. Great inter- and intra-subject variability in response existed for the normal speakers with no real learning effect occurring over the six trials.
2. Compared with Stromsta's normal speakers, the mean for the stutterers in the present study was significantly larger at 900 Hz only. Performance of the stutterers was significantly more variable at all frequencies except 300 Hz.
3. The means for Stromsta's stutterers were significantly larger than those for the stutterers in the present study at 1200 and 1800 Hz. The stutterers in the present study were significantly more variable at 600, 900, and 2400 Hz.
4. The mean differences between Trials 1 and 2 were not significant at any frequency for the stutterers in the present study.

Several factors were discussed which could contribute to the variability found in a study involving the cancellation process. Such factors included ambient noise levels, time requirements, movitation and concentration on the part of the listener, head and jaw movements, blood pressure changes, and type and placement of the bone oscillator. It was the experimenter's belief that the single most important factor contributing to the greater variability found in this study as compared with Stromsta's study was the type and/or placement of the bone oscillator. Findings of this study question the feasibility and reliability of using the cancellation process to establish a criterion measure for between-group comparisons.

### Kirkland, Wendy Rita, Oral Form Discrimination Abilities on Children Who Stutter, 1975.

A test of oral form discrimination, involving between-shape comparisons, was administered to twelve children who stutter and to twelve normal speaking children. Children in the two groups were paired on the basis of age and sex. The number of error responses and the mean length of time required to orally manipulate test items were determined for each child. Group comparisons were made using a $t$ test for related data.

The children who stutter made significantly more error responses than did the normal speaking children, thereby demonstrating a less effective oral tactile system. The children who stutter also required a significantly longer time to manipulate test items than did the normal speakers, possibly indicating less experience in using the oral feedback mechanism, as suggested by Gruber (1965) and Van Riper (1971).

The results of this study give limited support to Wingate's (1966) hypothesis that stuttering is an inability to make rapid articulatory transitions. Some support is also given to the hypothesis that may result from inadequate use of oral sensory feedback in monitoring speech. In view of these findings, assessment and training of the oral-tactile system may be an appropriate approach to stuttering therapy.

Children in both groups had difficulty discriminating the shapes that were similar. Easy items for both groups were those items that were most dissimilar in shape. Children in both groups responded "same" more often than was appropriate.

Future research in this area should include additional testing of both adults and children who stutter. Further definition of the exact of the exact nature of their oral tactile abilities is needed. The oral tactile abilities of adults who are recovered stutterers might be compared to the oral tactile abilities of adults who continue to stutter, because increased oral tactile might be one factor involved in recovery. Populations of children might be subdivided into specific groups such as "severe" and "mild" stutterers because children who stutter may not be a homogeneous group in regard to their oral tactile abilities.

**Koberlein, Susan Marie, The Phonological Consistency on Stuttering and the Frequency with which it Occurs on Function Versus Lexical Words in the Speech of Children Who Stutter, 1972.**

Three children with stuttered speech were tape recorded to obtain speech samples using three sets of stimuli. The stimulus materials included transformational sentence examples which the child was required to repeat after the examiner gave the stimulus, the expressive portion of the Northwestern Syntax Screening Test which required the child to respond after a delayed stimulus, and pictures from the Peabody Language Development kits used in combination with general stimulus questions designed to elicit as much spontaneous speech as possible.

Accurate transcripts were made of each child's speech sample and judged for disfluency. The criterion measure used to establish the sample of disfluencies for this study was judgment agreement by at least three out of the four judges. The data were analyzed to determine whether more stuttering occurs on lexical versus functional words in the speech of children who stutter. In addition, the data were analyzed for evidence of some common phonetic consistency. The results of this study were as follows:

1. Stuttering does occur more frequently on lexical words as opposed to function words in the speech of children who stutter. However, for the most part, the parts of speech appeared among the subjects' stuttered words about as often as they figured in the subjects' total output, especially in spontaneous speech. Only the conjunctions and pronouns contributed a greater proportion to the subjects' stuttered speech.

2. Analysis of those words subsequent to instances of stuttering shows that there was a consistently high frequency of occurrence of lexical words as opposed to function words.

3. The phonetic analysis shows that these three children do have some common phonetic elements that consistently occurred more frequently than the rest of the initial phonemes; however, this phonetic consistency cannot be universally applied to all children who stutter.

4. More stuttering was found to occur on words whose initial phonetic elements were:
   a) consonants as opposed to vowels,
   b) voiced as opposed to voiceless sounds,
   c) classified as postdentally produced, and
   d) those whose manner of production was described as fricative.

**Nahin, Melinda Joyce, Comparisons of Disfluencies for Voiced and Voiced-Voiceless Passages, 1980.**

The primary purpose of this study was to determine if stuttering subjects produce a significantly greater number of disfluencies while reading a passage containing voiced and voiceless consanants (Passable B) as opposed to a passage containing only voiced consonants (Passage A). A second purpose of the study was to determine if stutterers exhibit a significantly greater number of disfluencies on target words containing voiced and voiceless consonants as opposed to target words containing all voiced consonants. The target words were constructed in pairs so that in Passage B (containing voiced and voiceless consonants) each target word contained a voiceless cognate of a voiced consonant that was present in the target words of Passage A (containing only voiced consonants).

The sample consisted of 10 stutterers judged to be mild to severe stutterers. The age range was 18 to 42 years.

Each subject read two passages containing 279 words. Readings were separated by a period no less than one week. The order of the presentations of the passages was randomized.

Within the limits of this study the following conclusions are warranted:

1. The overall frequency of stuttering on the two passages did not differ significantly.

2. The frequency of stuttering with the initial words of each sentence excluded did not differ significantly for the two passages.

3. Significantly more stuttering occurred on target words containing a voiceless consonant than on target words in which all consonants were voiced.

Inspection of the data suggests the possibility that only a few stutterers are affected by the presence of voiceless consonants. Replication of this study with a larger sample is needed.

Further research should be conducted to determine relationships between the phonatory complexity and the frequency of stuttering for stuttering subjects. The contributions of psychological stress should also be explored in relation to aerodynamic and physiological disturbances occurring during the moment of stuttering.

### Barbaria, Lynn Marie, Oral Form Discrimination Abilities of Adults Who Stutter, 1978.

The oral perceptual abilities of adults who stuttered were compared with the oral perceptual abilities of normal speaking adults by a task of oral form discrimination. The speakers in the two groups were matched for sex and age within three years. The responses were analyzed for the number of errors and the mean time required to manipulate the forms. The mean number of errors and the total mean time required to manipulate the forms did not differ significantly between the stutterers and the normal speaking adults. The results indicated that the adults who stuttered did not demonstrate inferior oral perceptual skills. These results agreed with the findings of Jensen et al. (1975) but not with the findings of Class (1956).

Kirkland (1975), in a similar study, found that the oral perceptual abilities of children who stuttered were significantly poorer than children who were normal speakers. Since the stuttering children were not able to make many of the discriminations that the normal speaking children could make and that the stuttering adults could make, she suggested that stutterers as children may be delayed in developing oral perceptual abilities. By adulthood the oral perceptual abilities of stutterers may no longer be delayed. It was further suggested that poor oral perceptual abilities may be a basic causative factor for stuttering in children, but by adulthood, when their oral perceptual abilities were normal, factors such as learning would have to account for the continued stuttering dysfluencies.

The stimulus pairs in the study did not appear to be of equal difficulty. The majority of incorrect responses occurred when both stimulus items were within one category of shapes, such as circles, biconcaves and ovals, and shapes with points. The mixture of difficult and easy items may have masked any real differences between normal speakers and stutterers and explain in part the lack of agreement among Class (1956), Jensen et al. (1975) and this study.

Ten randomly selected pairs of forms were represented to the subjects for an indicator of reliability. The reliability was deemed satisfactory and was similar to the reliability found by Rengel et al. (1968) in a similar study. Greatest reliability occurred on the pairs of forms consisting of the same form presented twice or pairs of forms that were grossly dissimilar. Disagreement occurred only on the pairs of forms in which both forms were from the same category: circles, biconcaves and ovals, and shapes with points.

**Bennitt, Barbara Ann, The Performance of Fluent Speakers Versus Nonfluent Speakers on Certain Central Auditory Tasks, 1977.**

The purpose of this study was to compare performances of normal hearing fluent and nonfluent subjects on certain central auditory measures.

The measures used were the modified tone decay test, the staggered spondaic word test, the synthetic sentence identification-ispilateral competing message test, the synthetic sentence identification contralateral competing message test, and the acoustic or stapedial reflex test.

Examination of the data produced by this study indicate no difference in the performance of the fluent and nonfluent subjects. The measures which comprised the test batter in this study are generally those employed in clinical settings and are used either in screening or diagnostic procedures. Whether or not certain neurological differences are determined to exist in nonfluent speakers, their performance in this study would suggest that these tasks assess an aspect of neurological functioning not contingent upon the fluency of the subject.

As more central auditory nervous system evaluation measures are developed, further studies to determine the reliability and validity of these tests with nonfluent speakers may be warranted.

**Westmoreland, Mary Margaret, The Effects of Word Function and Phonemes on Disfluency in the Speech of Two Children, 1975.**

The purpose of this study was to determine the phonological consistency of stuttering in children, and to ascertain whether more stuttering occurred on lexical or function words in the speech of these children.

Speech samples consisting of 2196 words were obtained from two nine-year-old boys diagnosed as having moderately-severe stuttered speech. The children responded to three speaking situations: sentence repetition, sentence repetition with an imposed delay, and spontaneous conversation.

Written transcriptions of each child's sample were marked for instances of disfluencies and analyzed with regard to the loci of stuttering relating to grammatic function and phonetic elements. The data in this study suggest the following conclusions:

1. Both children stuttered more on lexical words than on function words.

2. The first speaker experienced more difficulty than the second speaker on function words, and the second speaker experienced greater difficulty on lexical words than the first speaker.

3. Both of the children in this study had a greater percentage of consonants involved in disfluent words than the percentage of vowels involved in disfluent words.

4. Both of the children used the same proportion of consonants (60%) and the same porportion of vowels (40%) in the total sample.

5. The first speaker experienced greatest difficulty with words containing /k/ and /i/, and the second speaker experienced greatest difficulty with words containing /o/, /n/, /tʃ/, /ʃ/, and /p/.

6. The second speaker was more disfluent on words with initial consonants than the first speaker, and the first speaker was more disfluent on words with initial vowels than the second speaker.

7. The first speaker experienced greatest difficulty on words beginning with /ae/, /I/, and /h/. The second speaker experience greatest difficulty on words beginning with /θ/, /k/, /ʃ/, /m/, /g/, and /r/.

**Shubach, Nancy K., Listeners' Evaluations of Stutterers and Nonstutterers' Fluent Oral Readings, 1976.**

Tape recorded samples of eight adult male stutterers and nine adult male nonstutterers, each reading two sentences fluently, were presented in random order to 28 untrained listeners. This experiment was then divided into two parts. The first involved judgments of speakers' rate, rhythm, and intonation, and an objective evaluation of stutterers' versus normal speakers' rates. At this time the listeners were not told that some of the speakers were stutterers. The second part involved identification of the stutterers versus normal speakers and the characteristic(s) associated with stuttering.

In the first part of the experiment, the listeners were asked to judge each speaker's rate as *fast, average,* or *slow;* rhythm as *smooth* or *choppy;* and intonation as *monotone, average,* or *exaggerated* without knowledge that some of the speakers were stutterers. The speech samples were also timed for the purpose of comparing objective reading rates of stutterers and nonstutterers. Based on the extent of agreement among the listeners, the speakers were classified as unequivocally deviant, equivocal, or unequivocally normal for the characteristics of rate, rhythm, and intonation. The conclusions from this part of the experiment were as follows:

1. For the characteristic of rate, when the categories of equivocal and unequivocally normal were combined, listeners perceived significantly more stutterers than nonstutterers as using deviant rate. However, when those speakers whose rates were judged equivocally and unequivocally deviant were combined, the number of stutterers and nonstutterers classified as having deviant rate did not differ significantly. Of the stutterers, five were judged unequivocally deviant, nonequivocally, and three unequivocally normal. Of the nonstutterers, one was judged unequivally deviant, three equivocally, and give unequivocally normal.

2. Measured objectively, the mean speaking rate of 3.19 syllables per second for the stutterers was significantly slower than the mean rate of 4.37 syllables per second for the nonstutterers ($t = 2.42$; $df = 15$; $p = 0.05$).

3. For the characteristic of rhythm, when the speakers who were judged equivocally and unequivocally normal were combined, listeners perceived a similar number of stutterers and nonstutterers as using deviant rhythm. In contrast, when the speakers judged as equivocal and unequivocally deviant were combined, listeners perceived significantly more stutterers than non-stutterers to be using deviant rhythm. Of the stutterers, one was judged unequivocally deviant, five equivocally, and two unequivocally normal. Of the nonstutterers, none were judged unequivocally deviant, one equivocally, and eight unequivocally normal.

4. For the third characteristic, intonation, when those speakers who were judged equivocally were combined with those judged unequivocally as normal, listeners perceived significantly more stutterers than nonstutterers as using deviant intonation. When the speakers judged equivocally and unequivocally deviant were combined, the number of stutterers and non-stutterers perceived as using deviant intonation were similar. Of the stutterers, four were judged unequivocally deviant, one equivocally, and three unequivocally normal. Of the nonstutterers, none were judged unequivocally deviant, two equivocally, and seven unequivocally normal.

In the second part of this experiment, the same speech samples, randomized a second time, were again presented to 29 untrained listeners (the original 28 plus one new listener) who were asked to identify the speakers as stutterers or normal speakers. If a listener judged a speaker as a stutterer, he/she was also asked to note the speech characteristic of rate, rhythm, intonation, other, or a combination of these which served as the determinant(s) of his/her judgment. On the basis of the extent of agreement among the listeners, the speakers were classified as having been judged unequivocally as stutterers, unequivocally as normal speakers, or equivocally. The results were as follows:

1. Agreement was unequivocal that three of the eight stutterers were stutterers. Agreement on two was equivocal. Agreement was unequivocal that three of the stutterers and all nine of the nonstutterers were normal speakers.

2. Based on unequivocal agreement only, the proportion of stutterers and nonstutterers identified as stutterers did not differ significantly. When speakers for whom agreement was equivocal were included, the number of stutterers so identified was significant.

3. No one speech characteristic emerged as "the determinant of stuttering." However, deviation in rate and rhythm, either alone or in combination with other characteristics, were cited more often than deviant intonation.

The entire experiment was repeated one week later with 22 of the original listeners in order to evaluate listener consistency. The results were as follows:

1. Listeners tended to be consistent in identifying speakers as either stutterers or nonstutterers on two trials. The number of listeners who made consistent judgments was significant for all but one speaker.

2. The number of changes in judgments about deviant rate, rhythm, and intonation associated with stuttering did not differ significantly. The means were 2.83, 2.95, and 2.73, for the three characteristics, respectively ($F = 0.11$; $df = 2.42$; $p = > 0.20$).

3. Changes in judgments about deviant rate, rhythm, and intonation associated with stuttering were not related ($W = 0.014$; $^2 = 0.625$; $df = 2$; $p > 0.20$).

# Appendix—I

# ANALYTICAL REVIEW OF "TO THE STUTTERER"

MORRIS VAL JONES AND ROBERT I. ALLEN

*A digest and statistical summary of the ideas expressed by 24 former stutterers in "To the Stutterer" indicates those concepts that are considered most useful to the stutterer.*

In September 1972 the Speech Foundation of America published a short booklet (113 pages) composed of personal advice to adult stutterers from 24 formerly severe stutterers. All of these authors are now or have been speech pathologists. They provided 37 basic thoughts or concepts.

We believe that the original manuscript is extremely interesting, but it failed to put the basic concepts regarding stuttering therapy in a form that can be easily digested by the reader. In the more complete breakdown, typical quotations are included to substantiate the basic concepts. Although Van Riper's contribution was a summarizing statement, his "basic concepts" are included in the tabulation that follows:

1. **Change your pattern of stuttering** (22 authors): "You must learn to substitute easy, slower, more related movements for rushed, tight, forced movements." James L. Aten

2. **Analyze your present pattern of stuttering** (19 authors): "You, as a stutterer, must study your speech patterns in order to become aware of the differences between stuttered and fluent speech." Margaret M. Neely

3. **Seek professional guidance** (13 authors): "Therapy for stutterers ordinarily requires having a competent speech therapist available as a guide, one who can share experiences with the stutterer throughout the course of therapy. The companionship of a competent speech therapist is usually essential for therapy success." Paul E. Czuchna

4. **It is your responsibility—your problem** (13 authors): "Do not forget that even though you went to the most knowledgeable expert in the country, the correction of stuttering is still a do-it-yourself project. Stuttering is your problem." Harold B. Starbuck

5. **Fear and/or anxiety as a cause or result** (12 authors): "For most of you, fear grew because of repeated failure and the resulting embarrassment over that failure. Your hope is that fear can be unlearned by handling hard words and situations better." James L. Aten

122

6. **Seek additional speaking situations—take public speaking** (12 authors): "...expand your speaking situations—and practice—until you can talk comfortably at any time you choose to speak." Dean E. Williams

7. **Accept less than perfection in speech and other aspects of life** (12 authors): "Don't waste your time and frustrate yourself by trying to speak with perfect fluency." Joseph G. Sheehan

8. **No pill, easy cure, or magic formula** (11 authors): "Perhaps you were hoping that at least one of these stuttering experts would have found a quick, easy, magical cure for your distressing disorder. Instead, it is quite evident that no such panacea exists..." Charles Van Riper

9. **Power of positive thinking—optimistic attitude** (11 authors): "One of the principles that I found of most value in changing my stuttering problem might be called constructive assertiveness." Harold L. Luper

10. **Change your feelings about your stuttering** (11 authors): "Your fundamental task is two-fold: alter your speech behavior, and bring about positive changes in your self-perceptions and feelings." Frederick P. Murray

11. **Always some residual of the problem** (10 authors): "Judging from my personal acquaintance...there is not one who would claim to be completely fluent at all times." Frederick P. Murray

12 **Be open—honest—advertise problem** (10 authors): "Let your stuttering be heard and seen rather than continue to conceal it by hurry and quiet." Gerald R. Moses

13. **Analyze feeling about stuttering and/or yourself** (10 authors): "You should begin by facing and describing those feelings and behaviors that make up your overall stuttering problem." J. David Williams

14. **Stutter on purpose—"negative practice"** (10 authors): "Stuttering on purpose or 'faking' at the beginning of a conversation might help you stutter less severely and less frequently throughout the rest of the conversation." William D. Trotter

15. **Do not avoid sounds, words, situations** (9 authors): "Above all, keep in mind that the less you struggle in your efforts not to stutter, and the less you avoid feared words and situations, the less you will stutter in the long run." J. David Williams

16. **There are no physical causes of stuttering** (5 authors): "Because you stutter, it doesn't mean you are biologically inferior or more neurotic than the next person." Joseph G. Sheehan

17. **Try to put the listener at ease** (4 authors): "One way to make your listener feel at ease about your stuttering is to tell an occasional joke about it." William D. Trotter

18. **Eliminate mannerisms, such as blinking, arm swinging, etc.** (3 authors): "You will seek to eliminate these behaviors (head or arm movements, eye blinking, body rigidity) by increasing your awareness of them and separating them from your attempts to talk." Gerald R. Moses

19. **Work for inner calm and self-confidence** (5 authors): "Only when you approximate inner balance with a healthy coordination of feelings and

action can you rid yourself of your stutter and ultimately achieve relaxed and spontaneous speech." Dominick A. Barbara

20. **The "rhythm" method is sometimes helpful** (3 authors): "Practice speaking in rhythm to a definite beat." Joseph G. Agnello

21. **Join groups of stutterers for self-help** (2 authors): "Form groups! In this way you can help each other. It will be much easier for you when you can find someone in whom you can confide and who understands your problem." Sol Adler

22. **Read aloud with listener present and/or tape recorder** (2 authors): "Use a mirror and a tape recorder to analyze yourself. . . . " J. David Williams

23. **Read professional literature about stuttering** (2 authors): "learn all about stuttering: read everything you can regarding this disorder; there is much literature available." Sol Adler

24. **Stutterers are not neurotic or emotionally disturbed** (2 authors): "Actually, persons who stutter seem to fall within the same range of physical and emotional characteristics as persons who do not stutter." Gerald R. Moses

Only one author expressed each of the following ideas:

25. Learn to adjust to fluency. — Don Emerick
26. Work on general relaxation. — Hugo Gregory
27. Use a masking noise provided by electronic equipment. — William Trotter.
28. Undergo psychotherapy to change your personality. — John Boland
29. Read stories which contain characters who stutter. — William Trotter
30. Learn to expect less response from the listener. — Dominick Barbara
31. Psychotherapy will not improve your speaking. — Spencer Brown
32. Use substitute words or phrases when needed. — Spenser Brown
33. You are not alone: there are over one million stutterers in the United States. — Joseph Sheehan
34. Hypnosis is only of temporary assistance. — Frederick Murray
35. Do motor planning in advance of speaking. — Harold Starbuck
36. Rehearse anticipated speaking situations. — James Aten
37. Get a friend to "take over" the talking when you have trouble. — Henry Freund

---

*The California Journal of Communicative Disorders,* 3(1):47–50, Summer, 1973.

# Appendix—J

## RESEARCH FINDINGS

### J. Woodruff Starkweather

Dr. C. Woodruff Starkweather published *Fluency and Stuttering* (1987), in which he reviews the literature about the nature of stuttering. Here are representative examples of his findings:

1. The syllabic repetitions that the layman identifies as stuttering are common to all stutterers (Wingate, 1964).

2. Prolongations of sounds beyond the normal duration are also common in stutterers (Van Riper, 1984).

3. Blockages and postural fixations of the airway occur in some stutterers (Van Riper, 1984).

4. Stutterers attempt to postpone, interrupt, escape from, or disguise the core behaviors by performing very many other behaviors (Wingate, 1964).

5. In some stutterers, clusters of behaviors seem to occur in sequence (Sheehan, 1974).

6. The amount of tension and forcing tends to increase with age (Bloodstein, 1960).

7. Stuttering children tend to recover spontaneously (Ingham, 1985).

8. Female stutterers are more likely to recover than male stutterers (Andrews et al., 1983).

9. When stuttering begins in the adult, the onset is usually sudden and associated with a traumatic event (Freund, 1966).

10. Both normal discontinuities and stuttering occur more often in stressful situations (Dixon, 1947).

11. Propositional speech yields more stuttering than does nonsense material (Eisenson and Horowitz, 1945).

12. Stutterers have more diseases of the respiratory system than do nonstutterers (Berry, 1938).

13. Despite much research, findings indicate that the biochemistry of stutterers seems to be the same as that of nonstutterers (Hill, 1954).

14. "Stuttering" has been observed in a few nonverbal activities requiring precise sequential coordination, such as playing of musical instruments (Froeschels, 1943).

15. Zimmerman (1980) has suggested that stuttering is a disorder of movement.

16. Stutterers are late in passing speech milestones, perform less well on language tests, and show three times as many articulation disorders as nonstutterers (Andrews et al., 1983).

17. The laryngeal events accompanying part-word repetitions are different from those accompanying prolongations (Conture, McCall, and Breuer, 1977).

18. The locus of disruptions in stuttering has wide individual variation, some are more laryngeal than others (Ford and Luper, 1975).

19. In their "fluent" speech, stutterers may move their speech mechanisms at a slower speed than do nonstutterers (Starkweather and Myers, 1978).

20. A predisposition to acquire stuttering can be genetically transmitted (Records, Ridd, and Kidd, 1976).

# INDEX

## A

Addicott, John, 55
Adler, Sol, 124
Aesop, 33
Agnello, Joseph G., 124
Ahlbach, John, 108
Air-flow techniques, 54–57
    benefits of use, 55, 56–57
    description, 55–57
    indications for use, 54–55
    problems with use, 57
Allen, Robert I., 122
Anderson, Virgil, vii
Andrews, 125, 126
Aristotle, 33
Aten, James L., 122, 124

## B

Barbara, Dominick A., 14, 81, 124
Barbaria, Lynn Marie, 117
Becker, Stephanie Kay, 114
Bennett, Arnold, 33
Bennitt, Barbara Ann, 118
Berry, 125
Bevan, Aneuran, 33
Bloodstein, Oliver, vii, 10, 13, 53, 82, 110, 125
Bluemel, C. S., 62, 74, 82
Boberg, Einer, 33, 82, 111
Boland, John, 124
Breuer, 126
Brown, Spencer, 124
Bryngelson, Bryng, 82
Busse, Michael, 111
Byrne, Claire, 110
Byrne, Renee, 82

## C

Cancellation technique
    master's thesis related to, 114–115
    use of, 66
Carlisle, Jack, 64
Carlisle, Jock, 33, 82
Carnegie, Dale, 72
Chapmand, Myfanwy, 82
Charles I, 33
Churchill, Winston, 33
Claudius, Emperor, 33
Cobb, 13
Coen, 87, 89, 91, 92
Cohen, Nancy, 111
Conture, Edward G., vii, 82, 126
Cooper, Eugene B., 15, 64, 82
Coriat, 13
Czuchna, Paul E., 122

## D

Dalton, Peggy, 82
Darley, Frederick, vii
Darwin, Charles, 33
Darwin, Erasmus, 33
Delayed Auditory Feedback, 54
Demosthenes, 33
Denhardt, 88, 89, 91, 92
Despert, 14
Discrimination abilities studies, master's thesis, 115, 117–118
Dixon, 125
Duncan, 14
Dysfluency (*see* Fluency and Stuttering)

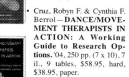

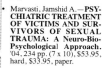
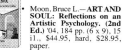
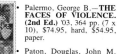
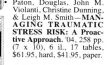
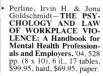
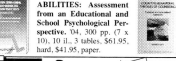
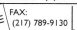

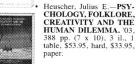
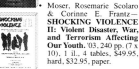

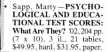
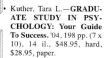
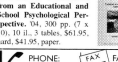
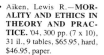
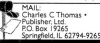